the Unofficial Guide™ to Coping with Menopause

Donna Howell with
Karen Brodman-Grimm, M.D.

Macmillan • USA

Macmillan General Reference USA
A Pearson Education Macmillan Company
1633 Broadway
New York, New York 10019-6785

ISBN: 0-02-862694-X

Manufactured in the United States of America

10 9 8 7 6 5 4 3 2 1

First edition

For Mom

Acknowledgments

The authors wish to thank Alpha Books publisher Kathy Nebenhaus and managing editor Jennifer Perillo for their help and their support while this book was being written. Also, thanks to my development editor, Nancy Gratton, my production editor, Kristi Hart, and my copyeditor, Kathy Simpson, for their skill in transforming this from manuscript to bound book. Appreciation is also extended to Nina Graybill and Jennifer Farthing for their able assistance in the launch of this book project.

Contents

The *Unofficial Guide* Reader's Bill of Rights

We Give You More Than the Official Line

Welcome to the *Unofficial Guide* series of Lifestyles titles—books that deliver critical, unbiased information that other books can't or won't reveal—*the inside scoop.* Our goal is to provide you with the *most accessible, useful* information and advice possible. The recommendations we offer in these pages are not influenced by the corporate line of any organization or industry; we give you the hard facts, whether those institutions like them or not. If something is ill-advised or will cause a loss of time and/or money, we'll give you ample warning. And if it is a worthwhile option, we'll let you know that, too.

Armed and Ready

Our hand-picked authors confidently and critically report on a wide range of topics that matter to smart readers like you. Our authors are passionate about their subjects, but have distanced themselves enough from them to help you be armed and protected, and help you make educated decisions as you go through your process. It is our intent that, from having read this book, you will avoid the pitfalls everyone else falls into and get it right the first time.

Don't be fooled by cheap imitations; this is the *genuine article Unofficial Guide* series from Macmillan Publishing. You may be familiar with our proven track record of the travel *Unofficial Guides*, which have more than three million copies in print. Each year thousands of travelers—new and old—are armed with a brand new, fully updated edition of the flagship *Unofficial Guide to Walt Disney World*, by Bob Sehlinger. It is our intention here to provide you with the same level of objective authority that Mr. Sehlinger does in his brainchild.

The Unofficial Panel of Experts

Every word in the lifestyle *Unofficial Guides* is intensively inspected by a team of three top professionals in their fields. These experts review the manuscript for factual accuracy, comprehensiveness, and an insider's determination as to whether the manuscript fulfills the credo in this Reader's Bill of Rights. In other words, our Panel ensures that you are, in fact, getting "the inside scoop."

Our Pledge

The authors, the editorial staff, and the Unofficial Panel of Experts assembled for *Unofficial Guides* are determined to lay out the most valuable alternatives available for our readers. This dictum means that our writers must be explicit, prescriptive, and above all, direct. We strive to be thorough and complete, but our goal is not necessarily to have the "most" or "all" of the information on a topic; this is not, after all, an encyclopedia. Our objective is to help you narrow down your options to the best of what is available, unbiased by affiliation with any industry or organization.

In each *Unofficial Guide* we give you:

- Comprehensive coverage of necessary and vital information
- Authoritative, rigidly fact-checked data
- The most up-to-date insights into trends
- Savvy, sophisticated writing that's also readable
- Sensible, applicable facts and secrets that only an insider knows

Special Features

Every book in our series offers the following six special sidebars in the margins that were devised to help you get things done cheaply, efficiently, and smartly.

1. "Timesaver"—tips and shortcuts that save you time.
2. "Moneysaver"—tips and shortcuts that save you money.
3. "Watch Out!"—more serious cautions and warnings.
4. "Bright Idea"—general tips and shortcuts to help you find an easier or smarter way to do something.
5. "Quote"—statements from real people that are intended to be prescriptive and valuable to you.
6. "Unofficially..."—an insider's fact or anecdote.

We also recognize your need to have quick information at your fingertips, and have thus provided the following comprehensive sections at the back of the book:

1. Glossary: Definitions of complicated terminology and jargon.
2. Resource Guide: Lists of relevant agencies,
   associations, institutions, Web sites, etc.
3. Recommended Reading List: Suggested titles
   that can help you get more in-depth information on related topics.
4. Index.

Letters, Comments, and Questions from Readers

We strive to continually improve the *Unofficial* series,
and input from our readers is a valuable way for us
to do that. Many of those who have used the
Unofficial Guide travel books write to the authors to
ask questions, make comments, or share their own
discoveries and lessons. For lifestyle *Unofficial
Guides,* we would also appreciate all such correspon-
dence, both positive and critical, and we will make
best efforts to incorporate appropriate readers'
feedback and comments in revised editions of this
work.

How to write to us:
Unofficial Guides
Macmillan Lifestyle Guides
Macmillan Publishing
1633 Broadway
New York, NY 10019
Attention: Reader's Comments

The *Unofficial Guide* Panel of Experts

The *Unofficial* editorial team recognizes that you've purchased this book with the expectation of getting the most authoritative, carefully inspected information currently available. Toward that end, on each and every title in this series, we have selected a minimum of three "official" experts comprising the "Unofficial Panel" who painstakingly review the manuscripts to ensure: factual accuracy of all data; inclusion of the most up-to-date and relevant information; and that, from an insider's perspective, the authors have armed you with all the necessary facts you need—but the institutions don't want you to know.

For *The Unofficial Guide to Coping with Menopause,* we are proud to introduce the following panel of experts:

> **Dr. David R. Allen, M.D.** is the founder of Integrative Medicine, Inc., bringing a fully integrated approach to health and healing. A graduate of U.C. Berkeley and U.C.L.A. Medical School, he studied internal medicine at Wadsworth Veterans Hospital and trained with

J. R. Worsley at the College of Traditional Chinese Medicine in England and the Hahnemann College of Homeopathy in Berkeley, California. He lives and practices medicine in Los Angeles, California.

Ada P. Kahn, Ph.D. is the author of *Stress-A-Z: A Sourcebook for Coping with Everyday Challenges* (1998). She co-authored several other books, including *The A-Z of Women's Sexuality* (1990), *Midlife Health: A Woman's Practical Guide to Feeling Good* (1989), *Menopause: Are the Best Years Ahead?* (1987), and *50 Ways to Cope with Menopause* (1994). Since 1994 she has been Manager of Community Health Education at the Rush North Shore Medical Center in Skokie, Illinois. She received her B.S. in journalism and a masters degree in public health, both from Northwestern University. She earned her Ph.D. in public health at The Union Institute, in Cincinnati.

Susan MacLaury, C.S.W., Ph.D. is an Assistant Professor of Health Education at Kean University in Union, New Jersey. She holds a masters degree in human sexuality, marriage, and family relations and a doctorate in health education from New York University, and her masters degree in social work from Hunter College School of Social Work. She has also completed two years of post masters training in clinical social work at Hunter College.

Introduction

W hen did you first start thinking about menopause? When your mother went through it? When you contemplated how many children you would like to have and your possible timetable? Are you still well in your childbearing years but experiencing changes known as *perimenopause?* Or have you found yourself around the age when many women approach menopause and only *now* are realizing that you too are going to cross that threshold, just as you crossed a threshold with your first adolescent menstrual period?

Back then, you may have talked about your first period with your mother or your girlfriends. Or the school nurse may have given you a kit with supplies and information. It was a rite of passage replete with promotional samples by the sanitary napkin manufacturers. To some extent you may have dreaded it, but you probably also looked forward to the changes it heralded.

What about menopause? The exact moment of *its* arrival is less clear to pinpoint than your first period. And what does *menopause* herald, really? Have you even talked about it with anyone? Do you know as much about it now as you did about menstruation when *that* began?

Actually today there *are* good sources of information about menopause available if you look, but no one's likely to take you aside, explain it, and hand you a menopause *kit,* for heaven's sake. So it will be up to you to seek out the advice you need and to formulate a philosophy of what's really happening with this change as your periods and fertility cease. You are older and presumably *wiser* now than when your periods began, so we're confident you can figure out this *menopause* thing, realize it is a *beginning* at least as much as an ending, and get on with things in good health and happiness.

This book was written to explain for you what's happening before, during, and after menopause. Since every woman experiences it differently, we've included ways for you to track your progress and resources where you can get in contact with other women to compare notes if you like. This is your body, and we hope you'll want to take a very active role in determining what's best for you, from finding an understanding physician who treats you properly to making decisions about hormone replacement therapy, herbal menopause supports, and alternative modalities.

We want to be very clear on one thing: Menopause is a natural change in your body, *not* a disease. In Part I, we'll give you the lowdown on *defining* menopause. Chapter 1 describes how it happens, how to know if you're approaching menopause and what to expect.

Chapter 2 provides real food for thought on the topic of menopause. Have you ever thought about *why* menopause occurs in nature? Rather than just designating the end of fertility, it seems to indicate a new phase of freedom for female humans and may also be a mechanism to ensure our health. You may be interested to find out about how some anthropologists view this important event in the life of a woman—some even suggest without it, the development of civilization might not have occurred as rapidly.

So, in Chapter 2, we'll take a look at menopause and menstruation as it's viewed in different cultures. In some Asian nations, for instance, postmenopausal women gain status and cultural approval to join in more day-to-day activities with males of the society. In Japan, women report far fewer discomforts as they progress through menopause than is common in the West. Part of the reason may be diet-related, and we'll give you a heads-up on that story later in the book.

In Chapter 3 we'll address the question: *What should you do about menopause?* The answer's different for every woman. For women who are experiencing some of the hallmarks of a less-than-trouble-free menopause (hot flashes, period irregularities, or mood swings) there is a range of options—from hormones to nonhormone drugs, to herbs, nutrient therapy, acupuncture, and other alternative treatments. If you're having a *relatively* easy time of it, there are still herbal supports, important nutrition and exercise programs, and stress reducers that can help ensure the rest of your passage is as trouble-free as possible.

You should never be too busy to make your own radiant health a top priority. With a typical woman's varied roles in life, from professional to wife to mother and whatever *else,* you may have to make a few adjustments to reduce stress levels, and you may have to find time for exercise, good nutrition, and for doing *those things that you find personally fulfilling.* At this time in particular, you need the support of good health without skimping on the important things.

Chapter 3 will show you how to take charge of your menopause experience. How do you find a good doctor, what should you look for? What kind of testing and costs may come into play? How can you research menopause issues that may affect you on your own? We believe that you should get all the information you can and make your own decisions. Say you're considering an estrogen patch. Talk to your doctor about the differences in brands and dosing schedules, and ask about what women notice when they use a patch instead of another method. If you're a computer user, fire up your Internet browser and check out some research studies on the efficacy of the patch, read up on its development, and most important, find a discussion list where you can ask other women about their experiences.

Part II addresses in detail how your hormones work, so you can get a thorough understanding of how their fluctuations may affect you. It begins with some important charting exercises so you can see a visual representation of your hormone-level cycles from menstruation to menstruation. Knowing how different hormones interact—and when—is vital if you're going to understand—and maybe even do something about—your symptoms.

Along the way, you'll learn some fascinating facts. For example, did you know that there are three *different* types of estrogen in the human female body, each with somewhat different actions from the others? And that there are many more less recognized types of estrogens that exert effects too? We'll delve into the way pregnancy and taking the Pill affect your hormone cycles during the month, and we'll explain what exactly happens to your cycle at menopause.

Next we'll deal with the problems that some women experience as their hormone levels decline—not always in sync—during *perimenopause.* Women in their 30s and 40s who experience more PMS than before, or less regular periods, and perhaps problems with infertility, may be navigating the tough terrain of perimenopause. In Chapter 5, we'll tell you how to determine if it's happening to you. And we'll detail what happens in the body when levels of estrogen, progesterone, and other hormones change, and explain why sometimes it's not the hormone levels themselves, but dramatic fluctuations in them, that can cause problems.

In Chapter 6 you'll learn about what happens after menopause. There are some major health concerns that you should know about, so you can take preventative steps. Osteoporosis, for instance, can occur if you've got insufficient estrogen, but you can take steps to ward off potential problems there, and there are also ways to monitor bone density, which we'll describe. Heart disease and certain types of cancers are also addressed.

In Part III we'll give you everything you need to know if you've been considering hormone replacement therapy. Chapter 7 provides some background on the history of hormone replacement. It hasn't had a trouble-free past, though many studies have led to refinements in protocols, and now there are a number of well-documented options for women.

We'll describe why progestins are often added with estrogen replacement therapy, what dosages are, and what timetables are followed through the month, and answer basic questions, like *will you get periods?*

When you're deciding with your physician about hormone replacement therapy, you have many choices. There are synthetic and natural hormones, different ratios of estrogen types, different dosages and schedules, and on top of that, you may have the choice of a pill, a patch, or even vaginally delivered hormones, or some combination.

Hormone replacement therapy is as much an art as it is a science, and the many variables it entails (that *delicate balance* theme again) makes it crucial to find a physician who you can really work with. You also need to know the risks involved—there are some, after all—and potential side benefits, such as help in warding off osteoporosis.

Chapter 8 tells you about *natural hormone replacement therapy* and how that differs from conventional hormone replacement therapy. Want to know about those over-the-counter natural hormone creams? You'll get a briefing on those products and other products, and we'll also tell you how to go about finding a pharmacy that can provide you with a natural hormone product, with your doctor's prescription. Not every pharmacy can fill the order.

Chapter 9 takes a look at new treatments coming down the pipeline—the so-called *designer hormones,* molecules that target specific hormonal tasks and that may avoid certain risks. Much progress has been made in this research area in recent years. Some women who declined to try hormone replacement therapy in the past because of contraindicated conditions may find that a designer hormone opens up that option to them.

But hormone replacement therapy, be it conventional, natural, or designer, isn't the be-all and end-all of options for support around menopause. Part Four talks about *treatments beyond hormones*. In Chapter 10, you'll find out about the latest scientific research results on specific nutritional therapies for menopause. You may know, for instance, that calcium can help prevent osteoporosis, but a new study suggests regular use of calcium (in the form of calcium carbonate) may dramatically reduce PMS symptoms—an important finding for women experiencing PMS and menstrual irregularity as part of perimenopause or menopause.

Chapter 11 covers some very important territory—how you can benefit your menopausal experience by adjusting your lifestyle. You'll find out how smoking and stress really affect how you go through menopause. You'll learn that it just makes plain old good sense to treat yourself well—if you take care of yourself, you'll make a positive difference in your menopausal experience.

In Chapter 12 we'll turn back to a consideration of conventional medicine, to look at nonhormonal pharmaceutical treatments that can help you cope with a difficult menopause. For example, certain antihypertensives (blood pressure medications) can help you cope with hot flashes, and there are some over-the-counter pain relievers and other medicines that may be just enough to ensure you're comfortable. You'll also find out which prescription drugs you may be taking for other medical conditions can have a detrimental effect on your hormone balance.

And you'll also learn some basic facts about *hysterectomy,* the surgical approach to very difficult menopause or perimenopause problems. It is an approach we hope you'll be able to avoid by educating yourself about the alternatives. But some women with severe gynecological problems may need to go to surgical extent for relief.

Part V introduces you to the alternative world of teas and supplements, folk remedies, and herbal medicine that's been used for centuries to treat menopause and its symptoms. Along with alternative therapies, you'll find out about where hormones show up unexpectedly in your environment—from the estrogenic soybean that may help you through menopause to the unintended and very different estrogenic chemicals present in some forms of pollution.

First we'll take a look at herbal therapies. While the use of herbs for a variety of ailments is only now gaining popularity in the United States, they're already widely used in some European countries.

Chapter 13 will tell you what you need to know about herbal remedies, from St. Johns Wort for menopause-related moodiness to Chinese patent formulas of many herbs (like the much-touted *dong quai* and *bupleurum*). We'll tell you which herbs are traditionally used for estrogen-support, which are for progesterone-support, and which may counter hot flashes, alleviate depression, and deflate bloating. And you'll learn about the possible adverse reactions and side effects some herbs can have. Just because something's natural does *not* mean it's safe for everyone in every situation.

Also in Chapter 13 we'll also take a look at homeopathy. Although conventional doctors frequently dismiss homeopathy as ineffective, it still enjoys a strong popularity, and many people swear by it. We'll tell you what you need to know so that you can decide for yourself. We'll also talk a little about acupuncture, which is now recognized by the National Institutes of Health as a useful tool in the treatment of a variety of conditions—including menopause. There are also forms of bodywork you may want to know about—such as *shiatsu,* an Asian form of massage that works along similar philosophical lines to acupuncture.

Chapter 14 deals with hormones all around you. Beginning with the *phytohormones* in foods, we'll tell you which edible is touted as having as much estrogen content as a typical prescription estrogen pill, and what common fruits and even grains can give you a little hormone boost. We'll also talk about hormones in meats and milk. It's a big controversy—should you worry about it? And we'll look at the effect of chemical pollutants on the hormone levels of animals—and humans—that come into contact with them.

It is our hope that, with this book, you will become better informed about your own menopause, carry away some positive thoughts about what menopause means in your own life and in society, and generally, that you'll realize you're *empowered* to cope with changes and succeed in living your life the best way you can. You have a lot of company in this experience—every woman in the world.

What Menopause Is

GET THE SCOOP ON...
What menopause is ▪ Common symptoms ▪
The female reproductive cycle ▪ Hormone
changes and health issues

PART I

What Is Menopause, and How Do I Know I've Got It?

Chapter 1

Menopause has probably been around since the dawn of womankind, although with the short life expectancies of early peoples, women often did not live long enough to experience it. The word *menopause* itself was coined a bit more than 120 years ago and ultimately derives from two Greek words: *mensis,* meaning *month* (and, by extension, *moon*), and *pausis*, from which we get our word *pause*. It and the time surrounding it is sometimes also called *the climacteric* (from the Greek word for *critical point*).

Most basically, menopause refers to that time in a woman's life when menstruation ceases—along with her capability to bear children. Today, we know that menopause can bring with it hormonal changes that have effects reaching far beyond the reproductive realm. A woman may become more skeletally fragile, her risk of heart disease may increase, she may suffer depression and loss of libido, and she may experience a host of other physical symptoms. And all this may happen *after* she's endured a year or two of hot flashes while her hormones learned to stabilize at their new, lower levels. (You can start having symptoms connected to menopause several years before your period ceases during what's called perimenopause, which we'll also address in this book.) In actuality, a host of hormone levels are declining throughout much of adulthood.

But none of these symptoms happens to every woman, everywhere in the world, in exactly the same way. Neither are they untreatable when they do occur. For some women, menopause simply means the end of an annoying monthly event—the menstrual period—as well as an end to the need for birth control. Menopause is a natural stage in your life. It most decidedly does *not* mean that your life is over, that you're becoming sexless, that you should feel old, or that you're physically deteriorating.

In this book, you learn all about menopause— what's normal, how to get through it with health and in comfort, and the problems that can arise. You also learn about the many ways that you can handle those problems, from the best approaches currently available through mainstream medicine to alternative treatments that have yielded demonstrable results. And we'll discuss *perimenopause,* which refers to the years before the actual onset of menopause. During this stage, smaller changes start to happen, and a woman can do the most to ensure her health for many vibrant years to come.

This chapter outlines the basics: when and how menopause occurs, its physical and emotional effects, and even *why* Mother Nature decided to do

Bright Idea
Your experience of menopause is affected by your general level of health. Eat healthy foods, and consider adding a high-quality supplement to your diet. More than two-thirds of Americans don't get enough vitamin E; more than half don't get enough A and B-6; and more than a quarter fail to get the recommended daily allowances of B-1 and B-2, C, and niacin.

things this way. Remember that menopause is a natural process that serves a legitimate biological purpose, and disease is not supposed to be part of the bargain. With reliable information to go on, you are in the best position to look out for your own health and happiness throughout this time of your life.

You may be menopausal if . . .

Menopause has long been blamed for any number of ills suffered by women when they reach a certain age . . . when their complaints weren't simply dismissed as being the rantings of a hysteric. (In fact, the word *hysteria* comes from the Greek word for the womb.) Depression? Must be caused by menopause. Irritability? Must be caused by menopause. Sometimes, menopause has indeed been to blame, but as we have learned more about menopause, it has become clear that problems which can be attributed to the hormonal shifts of menopause affect women of many ages—not just women of a certain limited age range.

So how do you know if you're going through or approaching "The Change"?

Menopause and perimenopause defined

Menopause does not occur as a single event. You aren't likely to wake up one day and suddenly discover that menopause has arrived. (If you do, and you have no other symptoms, you're atypical.)

The recognition of perimenopause—a new term in popular usage—reflects the medical community's realization that women's bodies tend to change gradually. A decline in the production of ovarian hormones can affect women in their 30s—particularly, perhaps, women who have never manufactured an especially abundant supply to begin with. A

Watch Out!
Smokers may experience perimenopausal symptoms earlier than nonsmokers do, even before age 35.

woman undergoing perimenopause difficulties has fluctuating hormone levels that lead to a confused menstrual calendar, or she may experience more subtle symptoms (see Chapter 5). Some medical schools of thought hold that perimeno-pause may be responsible for a number of maladies like osteoporosis and infertility, experienced by relatively young adult women (see Chapter 6).

Menopause is generally used to refer to that time in a woman's reproductive life cycle that leads up to, and includes, the complete cessation of menses. In fact, medically speaking, it refers only to that moment in time when menstruation stops once and for all as a result of a depletion of eggs from the ovaries, while perimenopause refers to the periods of time just before and just after that event. During this time, you may notice things happening to your body that are very different from what you're used to. For some women, the perimenopausal and menopausal period may last just a few months; for many women, it lasts a year or two; and for some it can last even longer.

The apex of menopause is when your period stops, but to understand what's really going on, biologically speaking, you have to look at *why* menstruation ceases. The end of menstruation involves a progressive decline in the functioning of your ovaries. Up until that time, your body was designed partly for pregnancy; during menopause, it gets a gentle (we hope) nudge to move on to other things.

Age ranges

The onset of menopause is determined largely by the productive life of your ovaries. This life cycle typically lasts approximately 35 years, but it can vary for individual women, as the following figure shows.

Timesaver
Start tracking your monthly cycle now, so that you'll have something to go on when you start to seriously examine menopause and perimenopause factors in your own life.

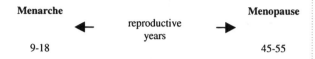

Menarche		Menopause
←	reproductive years	→
9-18		45-55

← Note!
A woman's reproductive years. This figure shows typical ages only. Health and other factors play a role in determining when fertility ceases. The most typical age for menarche is 12–13 years.

The natural cessation of menstruation that is the crux of menopause usually occurs when a woman is between 45 and 55 years of age; the average age of onset is 51. But menopause can begin as early as age 40 or as late as the late 50s and still be considered normal. The magic age for an individual woman to reach menopause is determined partly by heredity but is also affected by health and nutritional status. The better you're able to maintain a healthy lifestyle and diet, the later you're likely to commence menopause. You learn throughout this book about a range of factors that can influence onset age.

If you're a younger woman, take note: Menopause comes on prematurely (that is, before the age of 40) in about 8 percent of women. Early menopause can be induced when a woman's ovaries are removed or destroyed by X-rays or radium, and chemotherapy may induce early menopause in certain cases as well.

Common indications

For some women, the onset of menopause is relatively unmarked, but others may feel that they've suddenly stepped into the pages of a frightening mystery thriller. They experience hot flashes and night sweats, insomnia, a throbbing head, and emotional symptoms ranging from difficulty concentrating to panic attacks. It's amazing what a little hormonal fluctuation can do . . . sometimes.

Topping the list of well-known early physical symptoms of menopause is the hot flash. Sudden warmth and flushing begin at the chest and spread to the arms, neck, and face, often inspiring pleas to turn up the air-conditioning. Hot flashes usually enjoy three to six minutes of fame apiece, can occur several times a day, sometimes are accompanied by profuse sweating, and generally succeed in getting a woman's attention. Simply put, hot flashes can take a lot out of you. Fortunately, you *can* make these symptoms ease up, as you see in Chapter 12 and other chapters.

During a hot flash, many women also suffer pressure headaches, feel a bit nauseous, and have a tough time concentrating. The current theory is that hot flashes are something like overheating of your body, due to a sudden lack of the sex hormone estrogen. Another school of thought claims that this vasomotor instability (this fluctuation in the dilation of blood vessels, which causes many of these symptoms) is due not to the change in absolute levels of estrogen but to the relative shift in your body's production of estrogen from its previously normal levels.

Another common menopausal symptom—night sweats—may occur independently or may be associated with hot flashes. Both night sweats and hot flashes are frequently associated with insomnia. This situation can be doubly distressing. You are not only missing much-needed sleep, but are also likely to stay up all night thinking about the fact that you've probably entered perimenopause.

At the onset of menopause, some women also experience a drop in sex drive and begin to notice vaginal symptoms—specifically, vaginal dryness and the thinning and shrinking of the vaginal lining. These physical changes can make sex painful and can put a female at risk of vaginal and bladder infections.

Moneysaver
Maintaining a regular sleep–wake cycle goes a long way toward preventing insomnia. Bear in mind that your body responds to bright lights after dark (and during sleep) as though it were daytime. Try to keep light levels consistent with the time of day. You may be surprised how your body synchronizes. (In addition, this tactic is a cheap sleep aid.)

Finally, menstrual bleeding changes and may become irregular. Women often notice a decrease in flow and/or missed periods, and finally, menstruation just stops. On the way to period cessation, though, some women experience too much or too frequent bleeding. Although the amount of blood lost during a typical period isn't much, the change (particularly the increase) in its duration, combined with some or all of the other menopausal symptoms, can zap a woman's system and sense of well-being. Therefore, it's a good idea to try to stay healthy and do everything you can to give your body an easy time through this stage in your life.

As you'll see in Chapters 11 and 13, part of your basic strategy in counteracting the problems that can occur during menopause is to be as zen and untroubled as possible. Stress hormones make a big difference in how you experience menopause, after all, and they're always at your beck and call. The trick is to make a point *not* to call on these hormones, even if you have to rearrange your life a bit.

In some women, the emotional symptoms of menopause mimic premenstrual syndrome (PMS)—with good reason. Both conditions result from hormone fluctuations, such as a drop in estrogen levels. Some women find that they have reduced skin and muscle tone around menopause. These and other symptoms also may be chalked up to hormonal variations, not dissimilar to the problems many women have after they've given birth.

After childbirth the high hormonal levels (estrogen and progesterone) plummet. Many women experience emotional changes (known as postpartum blues), and if they decide to breast-feed, their estrogen levels remain suppressed and they enter a pseudo-menopausal state. The changes in the vagina and vulva at four to six weeks post partum are impressive and almost identical to the perimenopausal woman's experience. Many postpartum women also experience hot flashes

Following is a partial list of symptoms that are frequently associated with menopause:

- Irregular menstrual bleeding
- Hot flashes
- Night sweats
- Insomnia
- Vaginal dryness
- Vaginal and bladder infections
- Loss of libido
- Anxiety
- Depression
- Headaches
- Decreased skin tone

All these symptoms can be easily treated when it's recognized that they derive from the hormonal changes associated with menopause. Chapters 7, 8, and 9 devote considerable space to an exploration of hormone therapy—an important and still highly controversial issue. Part 4 examines other strategies that women have used to deal with the symptoms of menopause—strategies drawn from conventional Western medicine, nutrition, traditional Chinese medicine, homeopathy, herbs, exercise, and other methods.

If you're still wondering if you're menopausal, you can get the definitive word by asking a doctor to determine your hormone levels. But to assess the general likelihood that menopause has begun, try taking this little quiz:

QUIZ 1.1: COULD I BE GOING THROUGH MENOPAUSE?

1. My age is:
   (a) under 30
   (b) 30–35
   (c) 35–40
   (d) 40–45
   (e) 45–55
   (f) over 55

2. Close female relatives typically experience menopause as young as your current age.
   (a) Never
   (b) Infrequently
   (c) Sometimes
   (d) Often
   (e) Frequently
   (f) Always

3. I experience one or more of the following symptoms: hot flashes, menstrual irregularity, insomnia, night sweats, depression, anxiety, vaginal dryness, incontinence, decreased libido, and loss of skin and/or muscle tone.
   (a) Never
   (b) Infrequently
   (c) Sometimes
   (d) Often
   (e) Frequently
   (f) Always

Answers: If you answered nearly every question (e) or (f), you're a prime candidate for menopause. If most of your answers were (d), there's a reasonable chance that your symptoms are menopause-related. If you consistently answered (a), (b), or (c), you're probably not menopausal yet. But no matter what your answers were, any symptoms that you noted for question 3 could be linked to hormonal changes that can occur years before actual menopause, during perimenopause.

When and how menopause occurs

Your first inklings that menopause has begun appear as you enter the later portion of your reproductive life. Biologists suggest that the accompanying reduction in hormone levels may be a protective mechanism—the body's way of turning off the womb and its related gestational apparatus just at the time when carrying a fetus becomes riskier. But because the journey to a lower rate of hormone production tends to be gradual, the reduction in a woman's chances of pregnancy can precede by years the end to fertility that menopause brings.

Your reproductive life cycle from puberty through menopause

Watch Out!
Between 9 and 11 percent of menstruating women suffer iron-deficiency anemia. Prolonged or heavy periods, which sometimes occur as women approach menopause, can further drain iron stores. To reduce this problem, eat dark-green, leafy vegetables. Meats contain iron, too. A blood test can tell you if you're iron deficient, but be careful of supplementing any more than about 70mg a day without a doctor's orders.

Females are first introduced to the powerful role that sex hormones will play in their lives at about the age of 11. At this age, most girls start showing the physical changes of puberty, such as breast development and the growth of pubic and underarm hair. (Some girls, however, experience these changes as early as age 8 or 9 or as late as age 13 or 14.) The first menstrual period—an event called *the menarche*—isn't far away.

Just as women who are approaching menopause frequently experience erratic periods, adolescent females may also experience irregular periods during the first year. (The first true ovulation may not occur for a year or so.) The bodies of both menopausal adults and early adolescents are searching to stabilize appropriate hormone levels—a process that may take some time.

At puberty, cells in the ovary begin to secrete *estrogens*, which are the primary group of female sex hormones and which spur outwardly visible secondary sexual characteristics. The breasts begin to develop, for example, and the hips start to widen. Estrogens actually act on the bones to accomplish this widening, as the pelvis prepares to accommodate childbirth. At the same time, changes are taking place in the uterus and vagina as well.

But the secretion of estrogens doesn't tell the whole story. *Androgens,* which are secreted by the adrenal glands, are thought to be responsible for the growth spurt that adolescent girls undergo at puberty. Androgens (such as testosterone) typically are considered to be male hormones, but they are present and necessary (in careful balance) in the female body as well. When hormonal fluctuations start the countdown to menopause, the balance of androgens is often altered right along with the balance of the so-called female sex hormones—a situation that has its own effects. Chapter 4 provides specific details about the roles that these and other hormones play in menopause as well as in the menstrual cycle.

Thanks to the interplay of her hormones, a woman menstruates approximately every 28 days during her childbearing years—except, of course, during pregnancy and in some disease states. This monthly cycle is counted from the beginning of one menstrual period to the onset of the next. In the interim, a woman's body is preparing for two events: the release of an egg (ovulation), which usually occurs at midcycle, and pregnancy. If she is not impregnated at about the time of ovulation, the lining of the uterus breaks down and finally sloughs off during the next menstrual period, after which the process begins all over again.

During her peak reproductive years, a sexually active woman who uses no form of birth control has

Unofficially...
The age at which pregnancy becomes possible has dropped from about 16 to 18 years in the mid-1800s to the present average age of 11. This change is attributed largely to better health and nutrition.

a 15 percent to 25 percent chance of becoming pregnant during any given month. Fertility is usually highest during a woman's 20s, tapers downward during her 30s, and decreases further until menopause occurs during her late 40s or early 50s. After menopause, a woman is sterile.

JACKIE'S STORY

I didn't think about menopause. All of a sudden I just stopped having periods without any warning. I never had headaches, cramps, or other side effects. I was about 57 when I had the change and I felt great—no more messes! I had a baby when I was 41, late in my reproductive years, and I think that postponed it. I started menstruating later than most girls—when I was 16. That might be why I had menopause later on in life. Also, I know my grandmother had a baby at 40, and she stopped when she was older, too.

Though each woman's situation is unique, statistically the age at which menopause begins does not directly correlate with when a female experienced her first menstrual period. Neither does this age seem to be influenced by race, number of children, or use of oral contraceptives.

What's happening to me?

The female reproductive system is a marvel of feedback loops. If one hormone drops to a level that won't support the production and release of an egg during your monthly cycle, the fact that the egg has not been released affects other hormones, and so on. It's all a delicate balancing act. As the frequency of infertile cycles increases, so does the potential for perimenopause and menopause problems.

A woman may have regular monthly periods, yet actually be anovulatory at times—in other words, she may not be releasing an egg every month. A woman can begin to skip ovulations as early as her 30s, even though she continues to have periods well into middle age.

Along with experiencing anovulatory cycles, the body may become erratic in its production of estrogen and other hormones. Overly high estrogen levels may give rise to one set of symptoms, such as tenderness or bloating, whereas a sudden plunge in estrogen output to inordinately low levels can bring on other symptoms. Hot flashes are generally attributed to too little estrogen (although other factors come into play, as you see in Chapter 5). Table 1.1 shows a few typical symptoms of estrogen highs and lows.

TABLE 1.1: A FEW SYMPTOMS OF ESTROGEN HIGHS AND LOWS

High	Low
Breast swelling and tenderness	Reduced libido
Water retention, weight gain	Hot flashes, sweating
Mood swings, difficulty sleeping	Vaginal atrophy, vaginal dryness
Irregular bleeding (heavy periods) and spotting	Irregular bleeding (scanty periods)

As your body continues to wind down its reproductive clock, the changes in estrogen levels that affect ovulation can lead to irregular, missed, scanty, or unusually heavy periods. Essentially, your once-regular cycle becomes confused because the lack of ovulation affects your body's production of progesterone (literally, "pro-gestation"), a hormone that, after ovulation, readies the uterus to support pregnancy. If no impregnation occurs, your body's progesterone level drops off about 12 days after ovulation, and that decline is what spurs your period. But as menopause brings an end to your childbearing years, your hormone levels settle in at lower levels— ideally, with some synchrony. Your uterus no longer undergoes its monthly buildup in preparation for an egg release, you do not ovulate, and you have no proliferated lining to shed in a period every month.

Moneysaver
How can you tell if you're still ovulating without going to a doctor? Track your temperature every morning throughout your cycle; you usually notice an increase just after you release an egg. Remember that this method gives you only a rule-of-thumb measurement; see your physician for tests that can provide definitive results.

A woman with favorable genetics for endocrine balance who stays in top health may never notice her anovulations, and her system's resiliency may reduce her hormone levels toward menopause in a more balanced and less drastic manner than a less healthy or less genetically favored woman might experience.

Menopause and your health

As you might imagine, fluctuating hormone levels and their potential effects can wreak havoc with a woman's health. But by taking serious steps early on to improve and maintain your health, you can make a big difference in the ease with which you go through menopause. Remember that menopause is a natural stage in your reproductive life cycle—not an illness. The problems described thus far in this chapter are fairly commonly experiences for women who have a thorny time of menopause. But aside from changing your reproductive status and ending your need for birth control and attention to your menstrual cycle, menopause does not need to be a change "of life." There's no reason why you can't live as well and in the same manner that you did before.

If you're perimenopausal or even just entering menopause, remember that you may still be fertile. If you want to avoid the risk of pregnancy, birth control is still necessary. Some women who thought that their periods were lost to menopause have been surprised to find out that they failed to menstruate because they were pregnant.

Your attitude toward menopause makes a difference in how you experience it. Mood swings due to hormonal fluctuations aside, women who have positive feelings about going through this passage

Bright Idea
Some herbal therapies used in traditional Chinese medicine are purported to have endocrine-balancing qualities. Acupuncture, shiatsu massage, and yoga are also used toward the same ends. For more information about these methods, see chapters 12 and 13.

certainly have an easier time of it. Try to take an objective look at what this change means in your life. If you're having emotional difficulties, try to determine just how much of what you feel is due to a physical cause and how much is due to fear or anxiety about what menopause might mean. Parts 3 and 4 of this book describe some treatment options for dealing with both the physical and emotional bases of anxiety and depression.

Some women have a great attitude about the onset of menopause; they see it as being a positive change ("What? I never have to deal with a period again? Thank heaven!"). If you're having trouble maintaining your emotional balance, these are good people to associate with. Talk to other women who have been through menopause. You can even join an Internet newsgroup. Newsgroups often feature active, intelligent discussion on the topic, and knowing that you're not alone helps. Chapter 3 provides details on resources that you can tap into, online and otherwise.

Many women find that the realization of approaching menopause triggers reevaluation of their entire lives. There's nothing wrong with taking a retrospective view, but don't forget to look ahead as well. You still have a great deal of life ahead, and you want to enjoy it, not spend all your time rehashing your past. Besides, you have some important things to think about right now—in particular, your present and future health. Along with some of the difficulties that women experience *during* menopause, you may face difficulties *later,* and now is the time to take steps to avoid or minimize them. The following sections describe some of the health problems that postmenopausal women face; Chapter 6 discusses them more fully.

Watch Out!
If you still want to have a child and wonder where you are on the menopause timeline, consult your gynecologist now. Hormone tests can determine whether you're fertile, and hormone supplementation may help your efforts. You also need to know about the risks involved with pregnancy during your later reproductive years.

The fact that these health problems have been identified as occurring in menopausal and post-menopausal women, however, doesn't mean they are directly connected to menopause. Men frequently experience some of the same difficulties. The link with menopause *may* simply have to do with the changing hormone levels that are associated with aging in general.

Osteoporosis

Bone brittleness is a big contributor to the high rate of fractures among the elderly during falls. Loss of calcium makes the bones more fragile, and hormonal therapy may go a long way toward preventing osteoporosis (so will nutrition and exercise). New pharmaceuticals that target osteoporosis prevention have also been developed.

Following is a list of the major risk factors for developing osteoporosis:

- A history of osteoporosis in your family
- Advancing age (the older you are, the greater the risk)
- Caucasian and Asian descent
- A small frame or low body weight
- Smoking
- Lack of exercise
- Disease and medications (cortisone or thyroid hormone, for example)
- Early menopause (natural or surgically induced)

Heart disease

Heart disease is another potentially huge problem, for women as well as for men. Smoking, lack of exercise, and a high-fat diet are all believed to play a role

Moneysaver
Menopausal women have an increased need for both calcium and vitamin D. Some dietary supplements contain both. Sunlight is another good way to enrich your vitamin D stores for free (just remember to wear sunscreen).

in the development of heart disease. Hormone replacement therapy may reduce risk, but it has risks of its own. Estrogen is thought to contribute to an increase in HDL (the "good" cholesterol) and to provide other protection. The ways it helps protect against heart disease are still under study.

Colo-rectal cancer

Colo-rectal cancer is another ailment that women need to be aware of during their later years. The risk of developing this disease is thought to be reduced by hormone therapy. Good health habits, too, go a long way toward preventing this type of cancer. Smoking, a low-fiber diet, lack of exercise, and obesity are all risk factors.

Alzheimer's disease

Although the disease is not fully understood, the symptoms of Alzheimer's include memory loss and general senility. Hormone-replacement therapy has had dramatic protective effects in some studies; postmenopausal women who received it had 40 percent to 60 percent less likelihood of developing Alzheimer's disease.

Preventing and treating problems

The best way to prepare for menopause is to maintain great health. If you make sure that you have optimal nutrition, get a decent amount of exercise, and keep your stress level low, you stand an excellent chance of having a problem-free menopausal experience.

When women move beyond these basic precautions to hormone supplementation, things get cloudier. Estrogen, for example, is associated with breast cancer. Bear in mind that what estrogen does so well is help reproduction-related cells proliferate.

Watch Out!
Every year in this nation, the death rate of women from heart disease is 10 times higher than the death rate from breast cancer, although women have a greater fear of breast cancer.

Unofficially...
In traditional Chinese medicine, the term for menopause is *Yian Kui*. Both acupuncture and herbs are used to treat problems that arise or just to ensure a healthy passage. Research suggests that Western women experience more difficulties during menopause than Asian women do. See Chapter 13 for more on Asian medicine

A woman must weigh the potential benefits of extra estrogen against its potential drawbacks. Part 3 of this book is devoted to the ins and outs of hormone replacement.

Progesterone and other hormones may also be prescribed in hormone-replacement therapy. In fact, the term *hormone replacement therapy* (HRT) typically refers to therapies that include progesterone (or synthetic progestins); an estrogen-only regimen is simply called *estrogen replacement therapy* (ERT).

A rollicking debate is under way in medicine over which hormones are best in replacement therapy. The medical establishment continues to use estrogen-replacement as a therapeutic tool (with supplementation using synthetic progestins often too), but new claims are being made for the benefits of natural progesterone (and sometimes natural estrogens). There is plenty of disagreement about the roles that these hormones play in the female body. Part 3 of this book presents the different sides of this debate.

Nutrition, herbs, homeopathy, and other approaches are popularly used in the treatment of menopause difficulties as well, as you'll see in Part 4.

Why menopause happens

Menopause is something of an enigma, and not just for the women who go through it. Biologists maintain that human women are a bit of an anomaly because female members of other species don't go through menopause; rather, they tend to remain fertile. Why, then, must human females face an end to their childbearing years? Scientists point out that in most other species, offspring can care for themselves more quickly after birth than can human babies, who are dependent on a mother for an extended period. Menopause, and the sporadic infertility that can precede it, may serve to shield women from additional childbearing and child-rearing responsibilities at a time when it's best for her own health not to have that burden. In essence, menopause may be good for you.

Lower hormone levels during the postmeno-pausal years may in themselves provide protection against cancer and other diseases. Although millions of women have benefited greatly from hormone replacement, millions of others have decided not to go that route and handled menopause by other means.

Menopause, and its appropriate treatment hasn't all been figured out, so you need to know all the sides of the story, as well as how to work with your doctor, and then tackle this topic as your own scientist. The rest of this book can help you chart a comfortable course through your own peri-menopause and menopause, and find out what will work best and most safely for you.

Just the facts

- Menopause is a natural process—not a disease, but the cessation of a woman's monthly menstruation and fertility.

- The average age for menopause is between 45 and 55, although earlier and later onsets may still be normal.

- Women may begin experiencing hormonal fluctuations and their effects even in the years before menopause actually occurs.

- Irregular periods and missed ovulations are common before menstruation finally ceases.

GET THE SCOOP ON...
Theories explaining menopause ▪ Early medical
treatments ▪ Increased life span and menopause

Chapter 2

Evolving Eve

Women have been going through "The Change" as far back as scientists and historians can tell (whenever those historical women were fortunate to live long enough to experience it). How menopause, or *the climacteric,* is viewed—and, to some degree, how it happens—has also changed over the ages.

Early societies that lacked knowledge of science and medicine tended to view menstruation and other aspects of the female reproductive cycle as being mysterious and even dangerous. Until fairly recently, even Western-trained biologists and medical practitioners characterized menopause as being a sort of evolutionary oddity, tending to treat it as a pathological condition rather than a natural adaptation. More recent research has given rise to the theory that menopause actually provides humans an evolutionary advantage.

This chapter examines the variety of ways that human societies have dealt with menstruation and menopause. The chapter also briefly surveys the changing ways in which early Western medicine

Unofficially...
A whopping 80 percent of women are relieved to see the end of their periods, and most do not let menopause stop them from trying new or risky things, according to a survey. (Source: North American Menopause Society 1997 Menopause Survey [conducted by The Gallup Organization].)

attempted to handle menstrual and menopausal problems, as well as some of the related old wives' tales.

Biological reasons for menopause

Is menopause a mistake of nature? Is the hormone-production decline among menopausal women a sign of disease or entropy? Evolutionary biology has some encouraging words. One theory is that menopause and the changes leading up to it may help women live longer than men do—something that women have apparently been doing for a very long time.

Among centenarians worldwide, women outnumber men nine to one. In the United States, life expectancy at birth is about 79 years for women, compared with about 72 years for men. Records from 1900 show that women outlived men even then, and researchers who traced survival patterns back to the 1500s found that the same was likely to have been true for that era. According to those who have studied such statistics, Sweden was the first country to record national death rates, and its earliest records (for the period from 1751 to 1790) suggest the average life expectancy at birth was 33.7 years for males but 36.6 years for females. The following figure compares the trends.

Does a causal connection exist between longevity and the hormonal changes that lead to menopause? Given the relatively short life spans of humans during large portions of history, it's questionable how many women were lucky enough to even reach menopause (although they may have outlived their male counterparts anyway). Educator Evelyn S. Kessler notes in *Women: An Anthropological View*

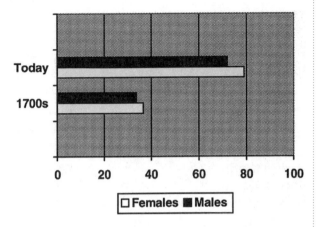

← Note!
Female and male
life spans.

(Holt, Rinehart, and Winston, 1972) that few societies take any particular ritual note of menopause. "In all probability," she says, "not many women in early societies lived long enough to achieve this stage."

Biblical references to life spans of several hundred years (literally to Methuselahic lengths; Methuselah reportedly lived to the ripe old age of 969) suggest that the incidence—and implications—of menopause were understood long ago. In the story of Abraham and Sarah, for example, the hitherto-barren Sarah is described as having her firstborn at the age of 90. Before the conception, God tells Abraham that Sarah will become "a mother of nations," but Abraham's response is to fall down laughing. (Sarah has a chuckle as well.) This story could imply that people may have routinely understood even then that menopause renders a woman incapable of conception, although the punch line may have more to do with Sarah's previous infertility than with the possibility that she was postmenopausal.

Theoretical explanations for menopause

Darwinian explanations for longer female survival relative to male survival are based on the assumption that the long-term survival of women is more important to the survival of the species in general. Interestingly enough, females *do* tend to outlive males in nearly all segments of the animal kingdom that have been studied.

Unofficially...
The sex hormones are thought to have evolved quite early in vertebrate history and have even been identified in invertebrates such as lobsters and starfish.

It seems that a life expectancy extending long after menopause distinguishes human females from females of the other primate species. The maximum life span for large-bodied apes is approximately 50 years, with fertility declining in accordance with other symptoms of physical decline. But human maximum life spans are about double that term, even though fertility typically ends right around the age of 50.

Rather than having biological importance primarily for the act of reproduction, the data suggests that species' life spans can be roughly correlated with the length of time that offspring remain dependent on parents, and particularly on the mother. In other words, researchers posit that it's not reproduction per se, but parenting, that determines life span.

Some anthropologists go a step further, suggesting that menopause figured in the development of civilization. One research team, headed by Dr. Kristen Hawkes of the University of Utah, conducted extensive studies of the Hadza people of Tanzania, and offered an interesting hypothesis. The Utah team's data suggests that postmenopausal women, freed from childbearing concerns, may have advanced civilization by helping rear the infants and children of other women, taking on workloads that younger women weren't able to handle. The data further suggests that grandmothers may have helped early humans develop new habitats.

Anthropological research has been critical of the trend in Western societies toward to the "medicalization" of menopause, that is, the presentation of menopause as a pathological condition warranting medical intervention, rather than a natural and perhaps evolutionary process.

It may be comforting to think that grandmotherliness could confer an evolutionary advantage on human society, but that theory still doesn't explain why a woman doesn't go on ovulating and menstruating throughout her life. One might easily think that menopause puts a damper on the transmission of a woman's genes to offspring, thus offsetting at least part of the argument for female longevity. In a June 1998 article in *Scientific American,* research physicians Thomas T. Perls and Ruth C. Fretts, instructors at Harvard University Medical School, suggest instead that menopause provides an evolutionary advantage by protecting females from increased mortality risk associated with childbirth at an advanced age (a woman in her 40s is 4 to 5 times more likely to die during childbirth than a 20-year-old is). Risks for the child are greater too. The following figure shows the risks of babies born to women in their latter childbearing years.

Menopause may protect a woman from the increasing health risk of pregnancy and childbirth. It may also be evolutionarily more efficient for a woman to ensure the survival of her existing children than for her to simply produce more—a reproductive strategy that potentially jeopardizes the welfare of the existing brood.

Note! ➡
Infant Mortality
Rate by Maternal
Age figures based
on research by
Friede, A.; Baldwin,
W.; Rhodes, P. H.;
Buehler, J. W.; and
Strauss, L. T.,
"Older Maternal
Age And Infant
Mortality in the
United States,"
*Obstetrics and
Gynecology,*
72(2):152-7 1988.
Fetal Deaths by
Maternal Age based
on research by
Fretts, R. C. and
Usher, R. H.,
"Causes Of Fetal
Death in Women
of Advanced
Maternal Age,"
*Obstetrics and
Gynecology,*
89(1):40-5 1997.

Infant Mortality Rate By Maternal Age
(compared to births to women 25-29)

Maternal Age	Infant Mortality
30-34	0% higher
35-39	18% higher
40-49	69% higher

Fetal Deaths By Maternal Age
(rates of unexplained fetal death)

Maternal Age	Fetal Death Rate Odds
<35	1 in 1000
35+	1 in 440

Although Perls and Fretts suggest that the edge in longevity that women have over men may be a byproduct of genetic forces related to childbearing and rearing, they make another interesting point. According to the Harvard instructors, males may live as long as they do (although admittedly not as long as females) so that males can pass longevity-assuring genes on to daughters, because of the evolutionary need for females to live a long time. In other words, the need for female longevity among humans could determine the life-span capacities of males and females alike. The theory is interesting, but like all theoretical reconstructions of early human society, it's not provable.

The search for insight, provable or not, into the potential hows and whys of life on this planet is a very valuable, if never-ending, quest. The possibility that menopause is a good idea for the species (as well as for individual women) adds a slightly different spin to the views of traditional Western medicine, which have sometimes focused more on treating menopause as if it were an illness.

Blessings or curses

Sex hormones are thought to be among the factors that both predispose men and women to, and protect them from, disease and aging. On the positive side, Perls and Fretts suggest that menstruation itself may contribute to the female gender's longevity by reducing the body's iron load, and also that the slower female metabolism may play a role.

But what about *andropause*, the still-controversial concept of male menopause? Some physicians and researchers characterize as andropause the gradual changes that take place in men as their sex-hormone production declines, as shown in the figure on the next page.

Some attribute reduced sexual desire, reduced potency, and increased urinary difficulties to andropause. Some also attribute the emotional changes of the male midlife crisis to andropause. These hormonal changes may occur during the same time frames that perimenopause and menopause occur in women. The male's testes produce less testosterone during this stage, just as a woman's ovaries eventually stop producing sufficient estrogen.

Clearly, neither gender is alone in producing a declining number of hormones with age. Men, however, have no physiological condition marking this decline that is as clear-cut as menopause is in women.

Myth, religion, superstition

Early cultures, and many non-Western societies of the present day, have treated menstruation as being an event of supernatural significance, to be dealt with by establishing taboos. Such taboos usually involve the seclusion of menstruating women from

> 66
>
> In my younger days, when I was pained by half-educated, loose, and inaccurate ways which we all had, I used to say, 'How much women need exact science.' But since I have known some workers in science who were not always true to the teachings of nature, who have loved self more than science, I have said, 'How much science needs women!'
> —Maria Mitchell, 19th-century astronomer
>
> 99

Note! ➜
Declining testos-
terone levels
in males. Graph
based on research
by Vermeulen, A.;
"Clinical Review
24: Androgens in
the Aging Male,"
*Journal of Clinical
Endocrinology and
Metabolism,*
73(2):221-4
1991 and
"Dehydroepiandro-
Sterone Sulfate
and Aging,"
*Annals of the New
York Academy of
Science,* 774:
121-7 1995.

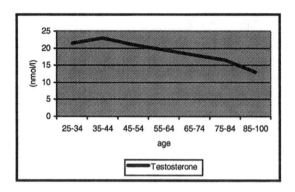

the rest of the society (certainly from the males) and frequently include elaborate rituals centering on the idea that menstrual blood is unclean or dangerous.

Sometimes, menstruation has even been described as being evil. Anthropologists, however, generally now attribute such strong terminology to prejudicial Western translations of local accounts of menstruation. Usually, only aberrant menstruation (excessively long or excessively copious periods) tended to be judged harshly—as proof in some cultures that the woman was a witch or possessed, for example.

In ancient Persian culture, menstration was said to last four days and woman spent their periods apart from society in isolated huts.

Women who were still menstrurating at the end of four days were whipped and sent back to their menstrual huts.

Anthropologists and historians can tell similarly eye-widening stories about cultures around the globe—enough to make one think that for at least some women of history, the end of menstruation must have been a blessed event.

Legends and lore have not dealt kindly with aging in women. We should be glad that life is not always a fairy tale because many fairy tales are (pardon the pun) rather grim. D. L. Ashliman, an educator at the University of Pittsburgh, writes, "The fear of oldsters (especially females) is further reflected in the fairy tales of many countries, where old women (even those who at first appear to be helpful and kindly) frequently turn out to be sinister witches" (*Aging and Death in Folklore*, University of Pittsburgh, 1997). That sentiment is clear in the stories of Cinderella, Snow White, Hansel and Gretel, and countless other fairy tales. Mother Goose herself is often pictured as being a craggy old woman.

Old wives and early doctors

Historians point out that the female reproductive cycle has not always been the domain of physicians. Throughout antiquity, doctors (who were almost always male) dealt mainly with disease, and the normal reproduction-related functions of the female body, ranging from childbirth and nursing to menstruation and menopause, fell to women—specifically, to midwives and wet nurses. These women frequently used herbal treatments to help their patients, and such treatments were often associated with magic.

Old wives' tales and treatments

The near-synchrony between a woman's monthly cycle and the movement of the moon in the sky was not lost on the Romans, whose goddess Diana was a fertility deity and later became known as the ruler of the moon, or on the early practitioners of herbalism. Supposedly magical cures associated with specific plants often depended on specific rituals, such as gathering the plants only by moonlight, when they were thought to carry the most power. Here are a few examples.

In Celtic cultures, the young maiden was seen as the flower; the mother, the fruit; the older woman, the seed. The role of the postmenopausal woman is to go forth and reseed the community with her concentrated kernel of truth and wisdom."
—C. Northrup, M.D., *Women's Bodies, Women's Wisdom* (Bantam Books, 1994). *See the Resource Directory in Appendix B for other books by Dr. Northrup*

Unofficially...
According to
Brad Steiger in
*Worlds Before Our
Own* (Berkeley
Publishing,
1979), ancient
Egyptians used
the equivalent of
contraceptive
gels and had
urine-based
pregnancy tests.

- St. John's wort, now popularly used for mood problems, was in folklore considered to be a potent way to attract love and happiness.

- Damiana, a herb that is purported to help regulate female cycles, was thought to have magical properties for inciting lust and producing visions.

- Ginseng, which is used in Chinese medicine for some menopausal complaints (among many other things), was considered to be a magic herb for love, beauty, protection, and even lust.

Old wives' tales about the properties of herbs (and the best ways to gather them) notwithstanding, herbs historically have played an important role in health care. Many modern drugs are derivatives of herbs. Aspirin, for example, comes from willow bark, which has been used as an analgesic for centuries.

Even some of the seemingly most preposterous old treatments have been at least partly validated by pharmacological science. Have you ever heard of Lydia Pinkham? In the late 1800s, she began making a treatment for women's ills, based on a formula that was purportedly given to her by a young Indian woman. This elixir contained herbs such as true unicorn root and pleurisy root, and had an 18 percent alcohol content (see figure on the next page). At that time, the beneficial effects of the compound were loudly debated, but Pinkham herself enjoyed a wide following among women, some of whom felt uncom-fortable consulting male doctors about their "female difficulties." Some ingredients of Pinkham's formula are still used today in herbal treatment of gynecological matters.

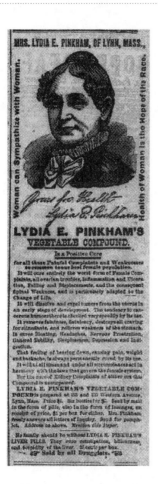

Women's issues and early medicine

Although woman-to-woman assistance is the historical rule, Hippocrates, the father of medicine, had
plenty to say about female ailments. Of menstruation, he wrote:

> If a woman is healthy, her blood flows like
> that from a sacrificial animal and it speedily
> coagulates. Those women who habitually
> menstruate for longer than four days and
> whose menses flow in great abundance, are
> delicate and their embryos are delicate and

waste away. But those women whose menstruation is less than three days or is meager, are robust, with a healthy complexion and a masculine appearance; yet they are not concerned about bearing children nor do they become pregnant.

Writing about classical health care in *Women's Life in Greece and Rome: A Source Book in Translation* (1992), Johns Hopkins University Press, researchers Mary R. Lefkowitz and Maureen B. Fant note that problems with a woman's organs were thought to affect the woman as a whole. Sexual intercourse and pregnancy were believed to help normalize difficulties. Beyond those remedies, the affected area was manipulated or medicines were applied inside the vagina, mainly to get rid of accumulated blood and fluids or to reposition an out-of-position uterus. Vegetable substances were used, as well as strong agents such as Spanish fly and even animal dung and urine.

Although early medical methods of treating women's ailments may seem to be barbaric, remember that the most popular estrogen-replacement therapy relies on extracts from the urine of pregnant mares. In that light, the practices of old are especially interesting.

Women are not entirely alone in their experience of declining sex hormones as a consequence of aging. History records the treatments used by men to handle their own age-related declining levels of androgens. The use of male sex hormones as a rejuvenating agent for men has been practiced since ancient times.

Animal testicles were consumed by men as a supposed aphrodisiac (and frankly, still are used for that purpose). Older men seeking the virility of youth later had testicular extracts injected into their bodies. And in the early 1900s, the sex glands of animals were actually transplanted into humans, with questionable results and often-horrible side effects. At about the same time, doctors even tried tying off the sperm ducts in the hope that by preventing the loss of sperm, they could stimulate the sex glands to make androgenic hormones that would turn back the male biological clock. The experiment didn't work.

Women's medicine in the early 20th century

Some modern women complain that a good bedside manner is difficult to find in a physician, and those who have felt patronized may find the words of an early 20th-century physician to be of interest. "The gynecologist looks after the diseases peculiar to women, and as a rule he is a very arrogant sort of fellow," stated Dr. John H. Tilden in his 1914 book *Diseases of Women and Easy Childbirth.* Tilden railed against the medical establishment of the day and favored natural approaches to healing. The health movement that followed his teachings, termed Tildenism, gained some popularity in its day, especially among women.

Tilden criticized specialists of the early 1900s for focusing on gynecological problems as being separate from the rest of a woman's physical condition. What affects the female sex organs, he reasoned, likely affects the entire body, the emotions, and the mind. Speaking of physicians of the day, Tilden wrote, "They . . . fall into the habit of forgetting that the female reproductive organs are a part of the body—that every organ or community of organs must be correlated with all the other organs to make up a body."

In his criticism of the medical community, Tilden anticipated the modern debate about whether too many hysterectomies are being performed when less drastic approaches would accomplish the same ends. Tilden wrote this about the medical community of the early 20th century: "The readiness with which they consent to sacrifice a part or all of an organ proves that they have a very loose idea of the community value of the various organs." He also said that thousands of women were "unsexed" in the name of "modern medical science" and claimed that "the reckless disregard of the consequences of mutilating women has been criminally great."

Although Tilden thought that gynecologists and surgeons were too quick to isolate women's gynecological problems from her overall health, he also criticized doctors for chalking up little-understood problems to menopause.

Tilden suggested that as many as 25 percent of the women of his day had fibroid tumors but didn't know it and never felt ill effects. He estimated that perhaps one case in a thousand really required surgery. It seems that not only fibroids, but also many other "female" conditions, were fodder for the early scalpel, as specialists sought to help in some way and responded in the only way that they knew. "The tendency has been for the past three decades to use surgery for the cure of all these diseases," Tilden wrote. "Why? Because of the inability to do anything else. It is cut or do nothing."

Was there a health-care utopia to be found despite the medical community's struggles to find "the right approach" to handling women's health issues? In Tilden's time, patient involvement appears to have been gaining a foothold, and among some, the old holistic ideas of Hippocrates were making a comeback. "Society is in a state of revolution, so far as doctors and patients are concerned," Tilden wrote, rather dramatically. "The brighter and more knowing slaves [patients] are repudiating their masters."

Menopause and the American woman

It has become widely assumed that American women (or at least Western women) face more difficulties, from hot flashes to missed periods to postmenopausal osteoporosis, during and after menopause than do women of some other lands. This belief, largely based on anecdotal evidence, has some support from the scientific community. Following are some scientific theories for the greater physical difficulties experienced by menopausal women in the West:

- **Chronic depletion of energy during childbearing years,** spurred by poor nutrition, stress, and relatively sedentary lifestyles. In Chinese medicine, persistent overstimulation of the body is said to lead to burnout of the "kidney essence" (which can beassociated with the Western alternative-medicine term "adrenal exhaustion").

- **The American diet,** which includes a large amount of animal protein. Some worry about the concentration of hormones in meat, especially because hormone supplementation of livestock has become a common way for farmers to enhance the profitability of their product. Hormone supplementation of livestock is banned in some parts of Europe.

Watch Out!
Enlargement of the uterus is most frequently caused by uterine fibroids. But new fibroid tumors don't start forming after the onset of menopause, and some existing fibroids may regress.

Moneysaver
Reducing stress is one way to help your body maintain balanced hormone levels through menopause. Don't overlook the value of this simple and largely free option.

- **Pesticides and chemical pollutants** that make their way into the food chain, water, and air.
- **Depletion of trace minerals** in the soil.
- **The effect of years of anovulatory cycles** due to excessive exercise (and the consequent loss of body fat), long-term use of contraceptive pills, or other factors.
- **The effect of prescription drugs** that are commonly used in the West.

No one knows for certain why women in some other cultures seem to have an easier time with menopause. The answer may involve not just environmental and cultural factors (including the typical diet) but also hereditary differences among and within human population groups around the world. But good nutrition, adequate exercise, and reduction of stress are likely to help ease the transition through menopause no matter where a woman lives and no matter what culture she's part of.

The importance of a culture's view of aging, youth, and (indirectly) beauty can have a major impact on the psychological consequences of menopause. In cultures that place great value on youth and beauty, the prospect of aging and losing a youthful appearance can be devastating. A woman's outlook on menopause can affect the intensity of her symptoms, as well as the psychological stress and anxiety that are associated with physical change.

"Changelings" in other cultures

Treatments for menopausal complaints vary around the world, from acupuncture and herbs in parts of Asia to the differing estrogen-replacement therapies of Europe versus those favored in the United States.

Traditional Chinese medicine treats menopause as being a normal occurrence in the aging process and describes aging itself as being a gradual depletion of Jing (Ching), which is the basic life essence. A traditional Chinese physician might describe the cessation of monthly bleeding as being the female body's way of conserving and redirecting this essence when the body can no longer prudently afford to use it for purposes of reproduction.

One of the "meno-puzzles" that researchers find is that women in non-Western cultures have significantly lower calcium intake than Western women do, yet they manage to escape high rates of menopausal symptoms, cancer, and hip fractures. These women typically ingest less animal protein (which can cause the body to excrete calcium and suppress the production of sex hormones). They eat more foods that are rich in potassium (vegetables, fruit, legumes, and grains) and are more physically active.

In Japan, for example, woman not only have fewer menopausal complaints, but also have an 80 percent lower rate of breast cancer. This fact has led some to extol the virtues of soy, a food that is high in natural estrogen, which Japanese women eat in much greater quantities than women do in the West. Although vegetarians must always take caution to eat enough protein, they may lose bone at just half the rate of regular meat eaters. In addition, vegetarians may need just half the calcium supplementation that meat eaters do.

Some cancers have a higher incidence in the United States than elsewhere. Relatively common cancers of the uterus, for example, which represent about 19 percent of all malignant diseases in

Unofficially...
In traditional Chinese medicine, the basic life essence is Jing (or Ching). The fundamental energy used in daily activities is known as Chi (sometimes written Qi). The spiritual and emotional energy of life is called Shen. Herbal tonics are used to enrich and harmonize these three so-called treasures.

American women, are relatively rare in Thailand, Japan, and Africa.

Replacement of hormones during menopause isn't strictly an American practice, but it's sometimes done differently elsewhere. The female body produces three main types of estrogen: estradiol, estriol, and estrone. In the United States, synthetic estradiol has been among the customary replacements for years, even though it has been proved to increase the size of estrogen-dependent tumors. European doctors are more likely to prescribe estriol, a relatively weak estrogen among the trio produced in the human body. Estriol is reported to help shrink estrogen-dependent tumors and to act as a protective agent against cancer.

Bear in mind, however, that established research on estriol is limited. Although some studies show that estriol fails to promote breast cancer in rats and may in fact protect rats from forming new breast cancers, the safety of estriol use has not been established by extensive studies.

Healthy emotions, healthy body

Part of getting through menopause swimmingly has to do with how you perceive it, and to that end, the definitions and observations attached to menopause and menstruation can be very interesting—even amusing. See if you can match the definitions in Quiz 2.1 with their source.

Thinking about your future

In the interest of ensuring women a smooth passage through menopause, researchers continue to look for new and improved treatments. Armed with new medical information pertaining to menopause, many physicians are taking an active role in treating

QUIZ 2.1: DEFINING MENOPAUSE?

1. "'Menopause' (female climacteric) is the final cessation of menstruation and therefore the end of a woman's reproductive life. The popular term 'change of life' is neither descriptive nor accurate, for it tends to indicate a physical, mental, and sexual deterioration, whereas deterioration does not occur."

2. "Menstrual blood . . . represents the essence of femininity."

3. "Hated something, likening it to "a menstrual rag."

4. " . . . only a woman can understand a woman's ills."

A. Simone de Beauvoir, in *The Second Sex*

B. The Biblical queen Esther

C. Lydia Pinkham, developer of an herbal formula for gynecological difficulties in the late 1800s

D. Encyclopedia Britannica

← Note!
Match the definitions and statements in the top section with the correct source from the bottom section.

Answers:

1. D

2. A

3. B

4. C

menopausal women and are reevaluating their approach to this phase of a woman's life. Alternative approaches are gaining credence and exposure, and women are increasingly taking it upon themselves to look out for their own well-being. The hope is that from all these approaches, the right preventive measures and treatments will arise.

Advances are being made. Even the duration of a woman's fertile years is no longer engraved in stone. In 1960, the average age of an American woman at the birth of her last child was 26.1 years; in recent years, fertility treatments have allowed women older than 60 to give birth. Fertility treatments that permit later-in-life pregnancies involve ovum donation, however, as well as in-vitro fertilization. Fertility with one's own eggs is not possible after menopause, it's thought.

A wise man ought to realize that health is his most valuable possession.
—Hippocrates

Chapter 3 discusses some trends in menopause care, as well as the foundation of good doctor-patient relationships.

Just the facts

- Researchers suggest that menopause may be a way of protecting the female from the burden of bearing more children, allowing her to care for existing offspring and pursue other interests.

- Extended care for offspring and long post-menopausal life spans make humans unique among primates.

- Hormonal changes at menopause may be partially responsible for longevity in females.

- The maximum age at which a woman can bear a child is no longer fixed. Through ovum donation and in-vitro fertilization, women have been able to give birth after age 60.

GET THE SCOOP ON...
Finding a great doctor ▪ Major menopause
health concerns ▪ Taking an active role

Here and Now

F or some women, menopause is as easy as waking up one day and finding that the awaited period hasn't arrived, and that's that. The monthly periods never show up again, even though these women's experiences of menopause have been very mild. If you're among the very lucky who notice no outward signs of menopause other than menstrual cessation, you can just go on as though nothing in your life has really changed. Right?

In a word, no. You may spend the rest of a very long and healthy life without having the problems that sometimes show up in the bodies of postmenopausal women, but an easy passage through menopause doesn't automatically guarantee you clear sailing in the years to come. Whether or not you're having difficulties now, take time to familiarize yourself with the conditions for which all postmenopausal women are at increased risk, and acquaint yourself with the most prudent ways to change your lifestyle and minimize your health risks.

This chapter outlines some basic lifestyle changes you can make, both during and after the onset of menopause, that go a long way toward improving the quality of your experience of this new time in your life. As you should with all health concerns, of course, you should begin by asking the advice of a physician who is competent in menopause-related health matters. But you should be prepared to take an active role in ensuring your own menopausal health. To help you do so, this chapter introduces some of the tools that you can use to research, share, and resolve menopause-related dilemmas whenever they arise.

It depends on your symptoms

During the past decade, there has been an explosion in information and medical options for menopausal women. In the past, a woman simply went through "the Change" and suffered. Occasionally, estrogen-replacement therapy was offered. Knowledge of perimenopausal women's health risks was limited. Luckily, interest in this phase of women's lives has grown exponentially. Medical research on diseases associated with menopause, treatment options for those diseases, the genetic risks of certain cancers, and the risks and benefits of hormone-replacement therapy are now high priorities, receiving funding and attention.

Menopausal women are no longer content to accept the changes that they are going through without investigating their options. The statement "It's not a hot flash, it's a power surge" says it all. Like a bolt of lightning, menopausal symptoms often shock women into actively managing their health. Women have become empowered and no longer accept changes lying down. Menopause is now a dynamic phase of many women's lives.

Once again, *menopause is not a disease.* As you read in Chapter 2, some researchers think that it may even be a survival mechanism, allowing females to concentrate their energies on caring for themselves and their existing families rather than on producing new babies. Although you may experience physical symptoms caused by the fluctuation of your body's hormone levels, these symptoms are not warnings of disease—simply your body's response to chemical changes, much like those that occur during puberty.

Defining normal menopause

In some parts of the world, normal menopause poses little difficulty, merely signifying the ending of a woman's season of fertility (and, thus, her periods). Nonetheless, despite making trips to the gym and taking daily multivitamin supplements, even the most health-conscious American women don't seem able to ameliorate all menopausal complaints. As a result, normal menopause, as commonly experienced by American women, includes hot flashes, headaches, mood swings, and the rest of the familiar complaints outlined in Chapter 1.

But the goal is to minimize, and even eliminate, the symptoms that may cause you problems. Step 1 toward achieving that goal is maintaining your health.

Health and fitness

Keeping healthy during normal menopause entails giving your body the nutrients, the rest, and the exercise that it needs to keep in balance. Staying healthy also requires preventive-medicine surveillance, such as mammograms, bone densitometry, sigmoidoscopy, pelvic exams, and routine medical evaluation by your internist. Everything from emotions to diet can affect delicate hormone levels, and as menopause approaches, ensuring that your lifestyle promotes equilibrium becomes especially important.

The issue of equilibrium is important. Before the onset of menopause, your body's hormone levels were relatively stable and resistant to disruption. During menopause, however, your hormonal levels are undergoing change, and they can more easily be thrown off balance by anything from faulty diet to excessive stress. Your first line of defense against unpleasant menopausal symptoms, then, may involve a change in lifestyle. Table 3.1 presents a few lifestyle tips that may help.

TABLE 3.1: KEEPING HEALTHY

Lifestyle Issue	Steps to Take
Stress	Reduce stress factors in your life, from relationships to your intake of stimulants such as caffeine. Take antistress measures: get restful sleep; try exercise, yoga, Tai Chi, meditation, massage therapy, and herbal and other nutrient destressors; and make time in your life for simple relaxation.
Nutrition	Quit smoking, curb your junkfood intake, focus on naturally healthy foods, watch your weight (but avoid fad diets), take a good multivitamin/multimineral supplement, and drink plenty of water. Also investigate herbal remedies or other specific nutrients that support female functions.
Exercise	Begin regular, moderate aerobic exercise for your whole system; and take up some form of weight-bearing exercise (such as running or walking) to improve bone health. Also consider doing stretching exercises (yoga, dance, and so on) to improve internal and external balance.

The difficulties that some women experience during menopause often have to do with lifestyle and, therefore, are preventable. Whether you're a woman in her 20s, 30s, or even 40s who is concerned with perimenopause, or whether you're a woman of menopausal age, now is the time to put your health first, to make sure that your body has the best resources with which to handle the passage.

Smoking is detrimental to your goal of minimizing menopausal symptoms—not only for the well-known health risks that it poses, but also because smoking decreases the effectiveness of the estrogen that your body makes. Women who smoke tend to go through menopause two to three years earlier than nonsmokers do. In addition, smokers are more likely to suffer from osteoporosis. So one of the smartest lifestyle choices that you can make right now is to quit smoking.

Pay attention to your nutritional needs, too. Now, more than ever, making sure that you're getting the recommended daily allowances of vitamins and minerals is important. Your comfort during menopause is directly related to your general health, and good nutrition is essential.

As for regular physical exercise, experts say that keeping fit and maintaining a normal, healthy body weight can help prevent or relieve many of the common discomforts that women experience during menopause. Regular exercise has the added benefit of helping prevent some of the serious health problems for which postmenopausal women are at increased risk. Exercise can cut your risk of (among other things):

Bright Idea
The American Heart Association publishes a guide to the risk factors involved in heart disease and stroke. The guide includes a section devoted to menopause. You can find the guide on the AHA Web site: http://www. americanheart.org/ Heart_and_Stroke_ A_Z_Guide/ menop.html.

- Heart disease
- Diabetes
- Lung disease
- Colon cancer
- Bowel cancer
- Lung cancer
- Breast cancer

Stress is a big factor in menopausal symptoms. Undue levels of stress—especially chronic stress—can strain the body by overactivating the hormones that figure into the "fight or flight" response, disrupting the delicate endocrine system that matters so much in maintaining your sex-hormone balance. Chronic stress tends to magnify small discomforts and decrease your body's capability to effectively deal with change. Stress also taxes your body's capability to deal with new challenges by monopolizing energy that could be better directed in more productive ways.

Defining problem menopause

More than three of every four women who are entering menopause experience hot flashes: sudden warmth in the face and upper body. Hot flashes (sometimes called *hot flushes*) typically last for a few seconds to a few minutes. Although minor hot flashes and similar symptoms need not be too distressing, for some women, the severity and duration can be so extreme as to be disabling. Other extreme symptoms include depression, insomnia, and severe discomfort related to the irregular occurrence of menstruation.

When a switch to a healthier lifestyle doesn't go far enough toward curbing such extreme symptoms, and when over-the-counter remedies aren't successful, many women turn to hormone-replacement therapy or other drug intervention on the advice of their physicians. Part 5 of this book provides details about the options in those categories.

How severe are your symptoms? Worksheet 3.1 lists some typical ones.

WORKSHEET 3.1: WHAT ARE MY SYMPTOMS?

Complaint	Mild, Moderate, or Severe	Chronic?	How Long?	Details
Hot flashes	_____	_____	_____	_____
Insomnia	_____	_____	_____	_____
Night sweats	_____	_____	_____	_____
Vaginal discomfort	_____	_____	_____	_____
Increased incidence of vaginal or urinary infection	_____	_____	_____	_____
Loss of libido	_____	_____	_____	_____
Irregular menstruation	_____	_____	_____	_____
Moodiness	_____	_____	_____	_____
Loss of skin tone	_____	_____	_____	_____

← Note!
Don't hesitate to seek your doctor's advice even for minor symptoms, which may indicate underlying problems.

Taking charge

You're already taking a proactive approach toward minimizing your own menopause-related discomfort by reading up on the subject. If you're just beginning to experience symptoms of perimenopause or menopause and your complaints are few, maybe all that you need to do is make a few lifestyle modifications. Changing your diet, stopping smoking, and getting a few weeks of regular exercise could yield the comfort that you need. Maybe you'll also consider taking an herbal or vitamin/mineral supplement. But if you've been dealing with severe problems that never seem to go away or have a solution, you may want to go further.

You should, of course, consult a physician who specializes in menopausal issues. But to remain proactive, you need to do some real research (hit not only the books, but also the medical journals, as well as the Internet newsgroups). You may also want to seek the advice of more than one specialist.

Even if your symptoms are mild and the physical changes associated with menopause are not an issue for you, now is the time in your life to assess your risk for certain health issues. Hormone-replacement therapy (or avoidance of hormone-replacement therapy) may be essential for your health at this time. *Not* investigating these issues is as important a decision as *investigating* them. What you do or do not do at this time, when decisions are possible, has an effect on your health and, thus, on your future.

Even if your menopausal experience is relatively easy, you're wise to research the long-term health issues of postmenopausal women. It's your future, after all, and forewarned is forearmed.

Remedy research

Many women have to search for their own answers in cases of difficult menopause. They may not find the right solutions through their first doctors and may try a variety of regimens before finding one that fits their needs. These regimens may include hormone-replacement therapy or the addition of herbs or nutrients to the diet. It helps, of course, to follow a healthy lifestyle and to minimize things that can further complicate a tough situation, such as stress.

Women who have had to go beyond their own physicians' offices in search of what works for them

Bright Idea
A simple word to the wise: Read up on something before you try it. Be careful always and skeptical when necessary.

need to find not only other women with whom they can compare notes, but also a doctor who will work with them on their own health care, listen to their suggestions, and offer good medical advice.

KELLIE'S STORY

Hi, everyone. My name is Kellie. I am 29 and had my complete hysterectomy in September 1997. Since then, I have been searching for the right HRT. I have had so many problems that I don't know how to deal with . . . insomnia, mood swings, hair thinning, joint pains, depression, stress, hot flashes (mild), and the list goes on and on! My life has just not been the same! I hate to blame it on surgical menopause, but I did not have these symptoms before my surgery. I am frustrated! Help! I look forward to getting answers with this list. Thanks, everyone!

At not even thirtysomething, Kellie had to embark on her own to find answers for a litany of difficult symptoms, and posted her message to an Internet mailing list to compare notes with other women. In a case such as Kellie's, researching menopause often becomes a preoccupation, even an avocation. Communication with other women who are willing to help and share comments is one way to get information on conventional as well as alternative therapies that may help. Sharing your story with people who have been there is invaluable as moral support, as well.

Whether your story is simpler than Kellie's or just as difficult, putting together the pieces of your own meno-puzzle means learning the skills of a researcher. Part of your journey toward finding therapies to make your menopausal experience easier involves getting behind the buzzwords and common conceptions to find out what's really going on. Where is new research challenging old protocols? What do women report about their experience with a product that claims to help? What are the

Watch Out!
"Complete hysterectomy" can be a confusing term, covering a number of surgical procedures, including: *Total Hysterectomy* (the removal of the uterus and cervix); *Subtotal Hysterectomy* (the removal of the uterus only); and *Total Hysterectomy with Bilateral Oophorectomy* (the removal of the uterus, cervix, and both ovaries). There's more information on the topic in Chapter 12.

dangers, as well as the benefits, of a treatment that you are considering?

The informal networking among women on menopause and hormone balancing "is a wonder to behold," notes John Lee, M.D., in *What Your Doctor May Not Tell You About Menopause*. There's nothing like word of mouth and hearing firsthand the experiences of other women who are going through menopause, each looking for answers to her own concerns and sharing anecdotes with other women.

Although you can research your menopause issues without a computer, the value of having one can't be overstated. Newsgroups, mailing lists, and message boards that have dedicated contributors—women just like you who want to share their research—abound these days. Medical journals are printed online, and at the very least, you get access to abstracts of their articles. Relevant essays and Web sites are a search-engine click away.

Table 3.2 lists basic useful sites for researching specific medical issues (menopause related or not) .

Note! ➜
Check Appendix B for an expanded list of Internet resources for menopause.

TABLE 3.2: GENERAL ONLINE HEALTH AND MEDICAL RESOURCES

Web Site	Description/URL
Medline search site	Provides access to medical journal abstracts through the National Library of Medicine's public search site for Medline http://www.ncbi.nlm.nih.gov/PubMed/
RxList	The Internet Drug Index http://www.rxlist.com/
CenterWatch	Listing service providing information related to clinical trials; designed as a resource for researchers and for patients who are interested in participating in clinical trials http://www.centerwatch.com

For the ambitious researcher who wants to find medical-study information herself and who isn't put off by advanced medical terminology, Medline is an invaluable resource for searching close to 4,000 professional medical and health journals. The bibliographic database is put together by the National Library of Medicine. Searching through PubMed, the public access site for Medline (http://www.ncbi.nlm.nih.gov/PubMed/), you can find abstracts on research and results. In some cases, you can get links to entire articles (for a fee).

How much can you really find out with a tool like Medline? A recent search on the term *menopause* retrieved 17,720 citations. A slightly more specific search, on *hot flash*, retrieved 36 study citations, dealing with such topics as the treatment of breast cancer survivors' hot flashes with vitamin E, relaxation-response training, and whether fever reduces the perceived severity of a hot flash.

Following is some of the data revealed by those studies:

- Researchers found that vitamin E produced a statistically significant (although clinically marginal) hot-flash reduction, compared with a placebo.

- Members of the Mind/Body Medical Institute (affiliated with the Harvard University Medical School) reported in *The Journal of Psychosomatic Obstetrics and Gynaecology* (1996) that daily elicitation of the relaxation response leads to significant reductions in hot-flash intensity.

- R. M. Barnard, F. Kronenberg, and J. A. Downey of the University of Michigan School of Nursing wrote in *Maturitas* that some women report fewer hot flashes when they have a fever.

Moneysaver
If you're new to online research and need access on the cheap, you may be pleasantly surprised to find that some public libraries and even coffeehouses offer free Internet access (and help). You can sign up for free e-mail accounts at sites such as www.yahoo.com and www.dejanews.com.

Bright Idea
The "Relaxation Response" is a simple method of meditative relaxation, described by Herbert Benson in his book, *The Relaxation Response*. (William Morrow Company, 1975).

An inquisitive woman researching menopause might ask how much vitamin E was used to get a "statistically significant (although clinically marginal)" response? Was this study done with huge loads of the vitamin or the amount that you might find in a daily multivitamin tablet? Access to the full journal articles can answer these questions.

In addition to offering articles that deal with menopause-related issues, several health-related Web sites have searchable databases, which allow you to find information on a specific topic easily.

Don't forget the message boards, where you can post a question to other women and read about their experiences. The newsgroup alt.support.menopause, for example, is an active, serious discussion center. You can also subscribe to private mailing lists that carry on lively exchanges.

Table 3.3 shows a number of Web sites and other online resources that deal in depth with menopause. Stop in for an overview of menopause issues as well as specifics.

Finding a great doctor

You are strongly advised to seek your physician's assistance with any difficulties that could be related to your passage through menopause. There's no replacement for the guidance of a highly trained, experienced medical practitioner. For all the proprietary knowledge that physicianhood entails, however, the profession is like any other, in that some doctors are dedicated practitioners who know a great deal, and others are not. Even among the real experts, you need to find a doctor with whom *you* feel comfortable. Part of your task as a prospective patient is finding the right doctor for you.

TABLE 3.3: ONLINE WEB SITES, NEWSGROUPS, AND MAILING LISTS ABOUT MENOPAUSE

Menopause Online
Advice and news on many menopause topics, as well as message boards and chat rooms
http://www.menopause-online.com/

National Women's Health Resource Center
National clearinghouse for women's health information and resources
http://www.healthywomen.org

Women's Health Interactive
Women's health site on menopause and other women's health issues
http://www.womens-health.com

Women's Health and Wellbeing WebRing
Web ring connecting sites about women's health
http://www.queendom.com/webring.html

OBGYN.net
Website on women's health for individuals and physicians
http://www.obgyn.net

Woman's Diagnostic Cyber
General women's health and gynecology site
http://www.wdxcyber.com

Doctor's Guide to the Internet
Internet site geared toward physicians, with section on menopause
http://www.pslgroup.com/MENOPAUSE.HTM

Mediconsult.com
In-depth site on medical topics, with section on women's health issues
http://www.mediconsult.com/women

continues

TABLE 3.3 *(CONTINUED)*

Midlife Passages
Comprehensive site on female and male menopause
http://www.midlife-passages.com

HotFlash!
Site on menopause and other women's health matters with email discussion group, chats, etc.
http://www.families-first.com/hotflash/index.htm

Power Surge
Online community for
menopausal women, featuring guest appearances by health professionals, chat rooms, and message boards
http://www.dearest.com

MENOPAUS List
Mailing list on menopause
(to subscribe, send email to listserv@maelstrom.stjohns.edu and in the body of the message put: subscribe menopause firstname lastname

menopause newsgroup
Usenet discussion group
alt.support.menopause

Curses
U.K.-based mailing list on menopause issues
http://www.tictac.demon.co.uk/curses/

How do you locate a good physician who can help you deal with menopause? The answer could be your current gynecologist or even your family doctor. If you haven't already broached the topic of menopause with either physician but have been satisfied up to now with the quality of their services and advice, make a point to discuss some of your concerns about menopause during your next visit, such as the ones in the following list. If you're looking for answers in the near term, there's no reason not to call for a telephone consultation about your menopause issues now, rather than wait until your next scheduled office visit.

- Decide whether you want to have a male or female doctor, and if you have a strong preference, gear your search accordingly.

- Make sure that the physician has board certification in his or her stated specialty (such as gynecology or reproductive endocrinology). Also make sure that the doctor's specialty fits your needs. If you have a serious underlying medical condition, such as diabetes, you may want to find a physician who subspecializes in that area.

- Speak with several physicians by phone before you decide who to visit. You can ask whether a free initial consultation is possible. Some doctors offer free consultations, and a conversation in person is often more relaxed and informative than a phone conversation.

You may not be completely happy with using your current health-care provider, however. You may prefer to consult a specialist if your menopause experiences are particularly difficult, or you may want someone who seems to be more sympathetic to

Timesaver
When you subscribe to an Internet mailing list, look for options that allow you to receive posts compiled in digest version rather than individually, to keep your e-mail inbox from being flooded with posts.

Bright Idea
Given the busy
nature of many
physicians'
offices, some-
times a brief,
polite fax
explaining your
inquiry and
requesting a
callback may
work best.

women's health issues than your regular doctor has been. In such a case, you can take the following steps to find the doctor who is best suited to your needs:

- **Ask around.** Quiz friends, relatives, and other associates for the names of physicians whom they know are good with women's medical issues. You can specifically ask for a gynecologist, if you want, but casting a broader net may get you more (and more interesting) responses.

- **Query your family doctor and gynecologist.** Either physician may know of colleagues who have particularly good reputations in dealing with menopause-related issues. It may help to make it clear that you don't want to switch doctors, just to get some outside input (about which you may be checking back with them anyhow). When querying your gynecologist, you may want to request a referral to a reproductive endocrinologist, an endocrinologist, or a specialist in osteoporosis, should your medical situation warrant specific expertise in a certain area.

- **Check your HMO/PPO specialist listings.** If you're a member of an HMO or PPO health-insurance plan, the list of practitioners may be limited. Your HMO plan may insist that you make an initial visit to your primary-care physician and receive a referral to a specialist or that you choose a specialist from a list. Look over your insurance policy and papers, and browse through your insurer's physician listings for gynecologists and endocrinologists. Also check under the headings "Women's" and "Obstetrics."

- **Check with a local women's clinic.** If you have serious budgetary concerns, contact your local Planned Parenthood clinic or another clinic that specializes in women's medical issues. These organizations may have physicians on staff who are adept with menopause-related concerns or may be able to direct you to other low-cost alternatives.

- **Call your local hospital.** Many hospitals have physician-referral lines.

- **Check with the appropriate licensing board.** You want to ensure that the doctor you're considering is board-certified (see Appendix B for board listings).

When you first meet with a prospective physician, you should have a well-thought-out list of questions. Following are some of the topics that you may want to cover:

- How many patients has the physician treated for menopause-related issues?

- Has the physician seen patients who have your particular complaints, and if so, how often?

- What is the physician's philosophy of treatment? Does he or she prefer to use hormone therapy or alternatives, including natural ones? (These kinds of questions are good for eliciting an answer that may give you real insight into the physician and his or her practice.

Look for a doctor who is board-certified. If you have an underlying illness in addition to your menopausal symptoms, you may want to find a doctor who subspecializes in that particular disorder. Also find out how long the doctor has been in practice. In addition, you may want to ask whether the

Timesaver
The headings under which women's clinics may be listed in your telephone directory vary from city to city. Check the following variations:

- Clinics

- Health

- Medical

- Physicians

- Social Service Organizations

- Women's Organizations

doctor offers a free consultation for prospective patients or requires them to make an official appointment.

Bright Idea
The National Institutes of Health is sponsoring a multi-year study of postmenopausal women. Among other goals, the study will explore the effects of diet, hormone-replacement therapy, calcium, and vitamin D on heart disease, cancer, and osteoporosis. Call the Women's Health Initiative at (800) 54-WOMEN or check out the organization's home page (http://www.nhlbi.nih.gov/nhlbi/whi1/) for more information about the study.

Additional questions to ask are who will see you if your regular doctor is out of town and which hospital(s) the doctor affiliated is with.

A word on handling disagreements with your physician: Among women and physicians alike, the challenge is to handle the disagreement and the exploration constructively rather than destructively. Although the medical community has made great strides in increasing its overall sensitivity to patient concerns, it is an unfortunate fact that some physicians still fail to see the need to work *with* their patients. These physicians may not explain why a particular therapy was chosen (or rejected) and refuse to listen to the patient's own observations or concerns. This situation is never acceptable. On the other hand, you, the patient, are responsible for respecting your doctor's training and expertise. If you are seeking your doctor's approval of "off-menu" treatments or therapies, you should be prepared to back up your requests with some research.

Avoiding problems, postmenopause

The decisions that you make about menopause now may have far-reaching effects throughout your life, and treatment is never a subject to take lightly. Following are some of the major postmenopausal risks and treatment concerns of which you should be aware:

- Heart disease
- Osteoporosis
- Breast cancer

- Colon cancer

- Potential health risks of hormone-replacement therapy

- Alzheimer's disease

Are you prepared to anticipate, and perhaps avoid, these risks? Take the following quiz to see how much you already know.

QUIZ 3.1: WHAT'S THE RISK?

1. Which disease accounts for 22 percent of all deaths among U.S. women?
   (a) Heart disease
   (b) Osteoporosis
   (c) Breast cancer
   (d) Colon cancer

2. Hormone-replacement therapy increases the risk of:
   (a) Heart disease
   (b) Osteoporosis
   (c) Breast cancer
   (d) Colon cancer

3. Hormone-replacement therapy decreases the risk of:
   (a) Heart disease
   (b) Osteoporosis
   (c) Breast cancer
   (d) Endometrial cancer

4. Which of the following conditions may lead to a problem that is more common than the risks of breast, uterine, and cervical cancer combined?
   (a) Heart disease
   (b) Osteoporosis
   (c) Endometrial cancer
   (d) Colon cancer

← Note!
Quiz Answers:
1 (a), 2 (c),
3 (a) and (b),
4 (b)

Here are some details regarding the correct answers to the quiz. Heart disease is the leading cause of death in postmenopausal women, and in the quiz above it's the appropriate answer to Question 1, accounting for 22 percent of deaths among women in the United States.

In answer to Questions 2 and 3 (Which of the diseases above may Hormone Replacement Therapy increase the risk of, and which may it decrease risk of?), HRT may increase the risk of breast and endometrial cancer while decreasing the risk of heart disease and hip fractures resulting from osteoporosis.

The answer to Question 4 is "osteoporosis," One-sixth of all women will suffer a hip fracture at some time, and these are more common than the risks of breast, uterine and cervical cancer combined.

Do the potential benefits of hormone-replacement therapy outweigh the risks for you? A test on the Internet is designed to help you decide. This test, which is based on individual health history, is on the Menopause Online Web site (http://www.menopause-online.com/hrttest/index.html).

Part 2 of this book discusses these risks in detail.

Treatment trends

As you search for the right way to handle your menopausal symptoms, take heart—new developments are in the pipeline. Following are some recent trends in the treatment of menopausal problems:

- Alternative methods of replacing hormones, such as transdermal patches, vaginal creams, and vaginal rings impregnated with hormones

Watch Out!
Watch your intake of foods that promote high cholesterol, and have your levels checked periodically. According to the American Heart Association, postmenopausal women show higher levels of triglycerides and cholesterol, very low-density lipoprotein (VLDL) cholesterol, and low-density lipoprotein (LDL) cholesterol than premenopausal women do.

- Selective estrogen-replacement modulators (so-called designer hormones) that target specific tasks in the body rather than acting as an estrogen on all estrogen receptors

- Hormone-replacement therapy provided in various proportions and sequences to suit individual symptoms

- Replacement of multiple hormones rather than just estrogen

- Replacement therapy that uses natural rather than synthetic hormones

- The use of herbs (combinations of Western and Chinese medicine)

- The use of specific nutritional supplements

- The use of foods that have hormonal properties, such as the estrogen-rich soybean, and the estrogen-supporting herbs red clover and sarsaparilla, or the progesterone-supporting chaste tree berry

- Yoga, acupuncture, Qi Gong (a method of energy manipulation), and other alternative treatments

- Regular exercise and stress reduction

- Nonhormonal drugs designed to prevent menopause-associated problems such as osteoporosis

As you find out more about these options, remember that your health is precious—and that it's your concern as well as your physician's. Be prudent in what you decide to try, and always consult your doctor first. Also look for other women with whom you can compare notes.

66

Because endings (whether musical resolutions, joke punchlines, desserts, or funeral eulogies) have a way of shaping the meaning of wholes—the meaning we attribute to old age shapes the very meaning of the entire human life cycle.
—Michael C. Kearl, professor of sociology and anthropology, Trinity University

Just the facts

- Watching stress, getting adequate nutrition, and exercising regularly are important to healthy menopause.

- Exercise can cut your risk of heart disease, diabetes, lung disease, breast cancer, colon cancer, bowel cancer, and lung cancer, among other diseases.

- The Internet offers active discussion among women about menopause.

- More than 75 percent of women who are entering menopause experience hot flashes.

- Taking an active role in managing health issues during menopause has long-term repercussions. *Not* taking an active role is in itself a decision and has its own implications.

How Your Hormones Work

GET THE SCOOP ON...
Sex hormones in the female cycle ▪
Monthly hormone-level fluctuations ▪
Tracking your cycles

Menstruation and You

Chapter 4

From your preteen or teenage days, when menstruation began, and throughout your fertile years, an intricate and delicate network of sex hormones has been humming away, following a nearly monthly cycle of ebb and flow, performing a balancing act worthy of awe. The interaction of these substances and the precise timing of that interaction affect not only whether and when you can conceive a baby or have your next period, but also a host of other things, ranging from your metabolism, your skin tone, and emotions to your sexual desire.

Understanding when and how sex hormones work in the female body is key to understanding perimenopause and menopause. In this chapter, you get the basics on the cycle itself, and you learn what happens to your body during all the major physical events of your life.

A day in the life of your cycle

Your menstrual cycle typically is 26 to 28 days long. Normal cycle length can vary between 24 to 35 days. Menstrual charting typically calculates day 1 as the

day when your menstrual period begins. By the time
your period ends, which can occur anywhere from
a few to several days later (the average length of
a period is about five days), your body has already
begun preparing for a potential pregnancy by stimulating the development of egg-holding sacs (called
follicles) in your ovaries. Meanwhile, the lining of
your uterus (your *endometrium*) thickens, storing
substances that will be needed to nourish a fetus if
conception takes place.

There are cycles and then there are cycles

There are several key points to keep in mind when
considering your menstrual cycle. The hallmark of
ovulatory monthly cycles (as compared to an interval
of time in which ovulation does *not* occur) is that
they are:

- Predictable in their timing. There can be some
  variation in the onset of the period but for the
  most part it is an expected event.

- Sometimes accompanied by mild premenstrual
  changes (medical terminology is *molimina*).
  These changes can include breast fullness, a little acne, mild cramping, slight moodiness, and
  slight bloating. (They are changes many women
  come to expect before a period.) These changes
  are the effect of *progesterone* production which is
  the hallmark of ovulation.

It is helpful to think of the menstrual cycle in two
phases. The pre-ovulation phase (follicular phase) is
dominated by increasing estrogen levels that peak at
the time of ovulation. Once ovulation occurs there
is a new player on board, progesterone, and it is *this*
hormone that is responsible for the symptoms associated with normal premenstrual changes. This

phase after ovulation (luteal phase) is dominated by high estrogen and high progesterone levels.

Menstrual cycle length is actually governed by the duration of the follicular phase of the cycle. It is this phase that will vary from woman to woman and will even typically change during a woman's lifetime, often with shortening of the cycle as a woman approaches menopause during the perimenopausal years. What remains constant during the normal menstrual cycle is the luteal phase. Once ovulation has occurred a menstrual period will start 14 days later. This remains a constant during the cycle (except in rare cases of luteal phase insufficiency). Once ovulation has occurred one of two events must occur: Either a period will begin 14 days later or it will not occur if the released egg gets fertilized (pregnancy).

This can be thought of in a different way: The normal menstrual cycle is actually two very different phases (follicular and luteal). The hormones governing these phases are responsible for the normal symptoms that occur. The event that separates the two phases is ovulation, and it is *only* with ovulation that progesterone is produced during the cycle. These are important concepts, and without understanding them, the changes that occur during perimenopause, when ovulation doesn't always occur reliably, will not make sense.

Eggs, ovaries, and ovulation

Ovulation—the release of a single egg from either the right or left ovary—usually occurs near the middle of the menstrual cycle. The egg travels through the Fallopian tube to the uterus. If fertilization doesn't occur, the endometrium, now nearly doubled in thickness, is shed (along with the unfertilized egg). This sloughing is menstrual bleeding.

The greatest number of eggs, or ovarian follicles (6–7 million), is present in us before our own births—when we're just at 20 weeks gestation!! From that time on the number of follicles in the ovaries decreases. By the time we're born only about 2 million follicles are present. By puberty the number of follicles has decreased even further to approximately 300,000.

Even though ovulation has not occurred yet, ovarian follicles are dying off and decreasing through atrophy. Thus at the time that ovulation starts an average woman has 300,000 potential eggs that can be released via ovulation. From puberty until menopause there is a gradual decline in eggs that is time dependent, with most of the decline being due to atrophy (aging of the egg cells). Most women will release one egg each month during their fertile years, with one of the following:

- An occasional spontaneous double ovulation (which may result in fraternal twins—unlike the chance splitting of a fertilized egg that will result in identical twins)

- An occasional induced multiple ovulation (via fertility drugs)

- An occasional anovulation (failure to ovulate) due to pregnancy, nursing, stress, or extreme weight loss

Most egg loss is *not* due to ovulation. Women who take oral contraceptive pills do not ovulate, but this will not cause a change in the time menopause occurs. Menopause occurs when the eggs in the ovaries become thoroughly depleted, as shown in Table 4.1.

TABLE 4.1: AGING AND YOUR EGGS

Age	Number of Ovarian Follicles
20 weeks gestation	6–7 million
Birth	2 million
Puberty	300,000
Menopause	depleted

The ovaries have two functions: They are the source of eggs, without which natural reproduction is impossible. (We can now bypass that with ovum donation—that's how 60-year-old postmenopausal women are able to get pregnant.) And ovaries are also a major source of hormones. The ovary produces not only estrogen and progesterone, but it also produces testosterone—in the part of the ovary between the follicles. Sometimes the extra hormones that stimulate the ovaries during perimenopause stimulate this area of the ovary as well. Many women find they suddenly have an increase in sex drive during this time due to the excess testosterone.

Roles of estrogen and progesterone

The synchrony of events during the menstrual cycle is governed in part by perhaps the best-known female sex hormones, estrogen and progesterone, with help from a supporting cast of other sex hormones.

Estrogen is the hormone that figures most prominently during the first half of the cycle, from shortly after your period ends until near the time that you ovulate. It can be produced by the ovary even if ovulation doesn't occur. Your estrogen levels peak shortly before ovulation. During this span of time, your ovaries—or, more specifically, the follicles around the eggs in your ovary—secrete estrogen, which spurs the lining of the uterus (the endometrium) to grow. For this reason, your uterine lining is said to be in the *proliferative phase*. When eggs atrophy to the point where they will no longer respond to stimulating hormones, estrogen production decreases and menopause occurs.

From ovulation until menstruation, progesterone takes an increasingly prominent role in the secretory phase of the cycle. *Progesterone* is secreted by the egg sac (follicle) after it releases an egg. At that point in its life, the follicle is known as the *corpus luteum* (Latin for *yellow body*). For that reason, the secretory phase is also known as the *luteal phase*. During perimenopause, a woman will have some cycles during which the egg fails to ovulate. When this happens there is an imbalance of hormones that may cause abnormal bleeding.

One of the roles of progesterone as it's being secreted from the corpus luteum is to signal the other ovary (the one that *didn't* release an egg) not to release an egg, in a neat check-and-balance effect so that multiple eggs aren't released during a cycle *(usually)*. Also, progesterone is sometimes called the pregnancy hormone because it is literally *progestational*—that is, it prepares the endometrium to support life should fertilization occur, sustaining the endometrial growth that estrogen spurred, and also inhibiting muscular contractions of the uterus that might otherwise cause it to reject a fertilized egg.

Levels of both estrogen and progesterone drop dramatically as the menstrual period approaches. The following figure shows when estrogen and progesterone levels typically peak during the cycle.

The female body actually produces many types of estrogen, which are sometimes referred to in

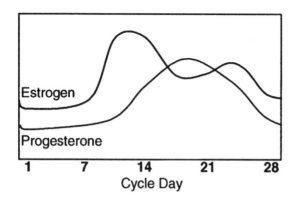

← Note!
These peaks and valleys are for a typical cycle during which a woman is ovulating. Levels can vary during cycles in which a woman fails to ovulate.

the plural, as *estrogens*. The three main human estrogens—estrone, estriol, and estradiol—are produced mainly in the ovaries of fertile women. Fat, muscle, and other types of cells also can generate estrogens, however, and after menopause, these sites become increasingly important to the body's overall supply of the hormones.

Table 4.2 describes the three major estrogens.

TABLE 4.2: THE ESTROGENS

Estrogen	Description
Estradiol	The most potent human estrogen
Estrone	A weaker estrogen, a metabolite of estradiol
Estriol	The weakest of the three estrogens, also a metabolite of estradiol

One important and interesting point about estrogen is peripheral conversion of estrogen that occurs in the fat tissues of the female body. What this means is that estrogen is actually transformed from other precursor hormones in the fatty tissues. Hormones from the ovaries and adrenal glands (testosterone and androstenedione) can be metabolized in fat and turned into estradiol and estrone. This is the reason heavy and obese women usually have fewer menopausal symptoms than thin women. The higher levels of estrogen (without a balancing amount of progesterone) can also put them at higher risk of developing endometrial cancer.

Progesterone, which is primarily made by the ovary's corpus luteum, is also produced by the adrenal glands of both men and women, and to some extent by the male's testes. Progesterone can also be turned into estrogen or testosterone (and some other hormones) by the body. Sex hormones are a tightly knit, if versatile, family. If it weren't for estrogen, ovulation wouldn't be possible, and the egg sac wouldn't be available for the production of progesterone.

Stimulating the Cycle: FSH and LH

Although you hear most about estrogen and progesterone, these hormones don't tell the full story of the reproductive cycle. Among the other important players are *gonadotropic follicle-stimulating hormone (FSH) and luteinizing hormone (LH)*. These hormones help determine how estrogen and progesterone are produced. Both hormones are secreted by the brain, in the anterior pituitary, and both act as messengers to stimulate the follicles of the ovary to function.

At the beginning of a new menstrual cycle estrogen levels are low. The receptors in the pituitary gland are sensitive to estrogen levels and respond by producing FSH. (This interplay of hormone activity where a lack of one hormone promotes the production of another is called *positive feedback*.) The brain in essence realizes there is not enough estrogen on board, so it sends its messenger, FSH, to stimulate the ovary to make estrogen. FSH stimulates a group of follicles in the ovary to start growing. It is these follicles that produce the surge of estrogen that characterizes the first half, or follicular phase, of the cycle. This is the first important duty of the ovarian follicles—to produce estrogen. As the estrogen levels increase the pituitary gland is able to detect that there is adequate estrogen on board and the level of FSH production is decreased. (This interplay of hormone activity is called *negative feedback.*)

As the FSH levels decrease the pituitary starts to manufacture the next messenger, LH. The following figure shows how FSH and LH fit into the monthly cycle.

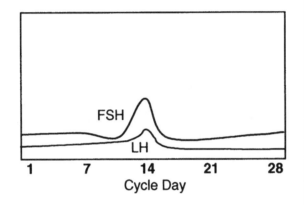

← Note!
FSH and LH levels fluctuate through the month.

At this point there are typically several follicles in the ovary that have been stimulated to grow. One follicle ultimately becomes the largest, or dominant, follicle. It is this follicle that is destined to ovulate with the proper stimulation, namely LH. As LH peaks at midcycle the dominant follicle ruptures and releases its egg. The ovary has now performed its second duty—to produce an egg. The fluid within the dominant follicle gets released into the abdominal cavity. Many women are able to detect the cramping sensation caused by this midcycle event. The medical word for this is *mittleschmertz* which is German for "middle pain."

After ovulation occurs, the ruptured follicle turns into a hormone producing "machine." In addition to estrogen it starts to produce progesterone. The increasing progesterone levels turn off the production of LH in the pituitary, and these levels return to baseline. The hormone producing "machine" in the ovary is called a "corpus luteum." If the released egg is not fertilized, the corpus luteum's life is limited to 14 days and progesterone levels decline. It is the decline in progesterone that causes the lining of the uterus to slough off, which is what a menstrual period is.

There are several changes that occur in a woman's body during the menstrual cycle that can be directly related to the above events. Understanding these changes will let you get a handle on your body's normal functioning if you are still ovulating and will help you identify changes if you are perimenopausal or menopausal.

Be aware of changes in your cervical mucus. The cervix is the opening of the uterus that protrudes into the vagina. The cervix has glands that respond to the fluctuations in hormone levels. At midcycle, just prior to ovulation there is production of mucus that has the consistency of egg whites. This is the effect of high levels of estrogen. Once ovulation occurs this mucus becomes thick and loses its characteristic consistency. You may notice this clear mucus for example when you wipe yourself after urinating. (As a gynecologist the appearance of this clear mucus is a sign that estrogen levels are not in the menopausal range.)

Identifying this characteristic clear mucus can be a clue that you are probably producing adequate estrogen levels and is a reassuring sign to those concerned about being menopausal. In addition, there are other signs to be aware of:

- Be aware of signs of *mittleschmertz*. It can be useful in making sense of the changes occurring in your body.

- Premenstrual symptoms are another sign of ovulation. These symptoms are generally the effects of progesterone.

- Body temperature will typically increase by one degree after ovulation. This is also an effect of progesterone.

Testosterone, which is commonly considered to be a "male" hormone, is also produced in small amounts by the ovaries.

Other sex hormones can come into play when dealing with difficulties during menopause. You'll learn more about their role in Chapter 5. In addition, levels of other kinds of hormones, such as thyroid, also affect a woman's overall health.

Other hormones

Progesterone and estrogen are but two of many steroidal hormones that get their start as cholesterol. A steroid is a basic group of structurally similar molecules that all start out with the same shaped building block. This basic structure is then modified in different parts of the body (the liver, ovaries, fat, adrenal glands) via chemical reactions to form the various steroid hormones. They are thus all "kissing cousins" so to speak. The molecules are converted from largest in size (cholesterol) to progressively smaller structures.

Pregnenolone, the precursor of all other steroid hormones, is synthesized from cholesterol. Progesterone is converted from pregnenolone and

Note! ➡
Not all the hormones that are part of the synthesis pathway are specifically sex hormones, although in some cases, sex hormones can be made from them, as indicated by arrows.

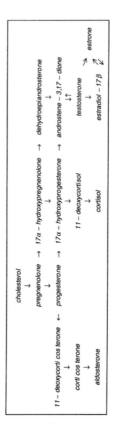

becomes a precursor to many other hormones, including the estrogens. *Androstenedione* and *androstenediol* are androgenic (male) hormones, although they occur in females as well. Both estrogen and testosterone can be made from these hormones.

Are they just sex hormones?
As hormone levels fluctuate during the month, they exert on the female body a wide range of powerful effects that fall outside the direct realm of reproduction. Progesterone, for example, helps raise body temperature at about the time of ovulation, thereby having a systemic effect, and estrogen affects blood pressure, among other things.

The balance of the sex hormones and the entire endocrine system can have a potential impact on a woman's current health and future risks, ranging from various types of cancers to cardiovascular disease and osteoporosis. The Population Council, an organization that focuses on reproductive issues, pointed out in a 1996 news release that wide gaps exist in research on links between the menstrual cycle and other physiologic systems.

"The menstrual cycle appears to modulate several aspects of women's physiology, including heart rate, pulse transit time and blood pressure, energy metabolism, and various aspects of immune function," says Dr. Sioban Harlow, an epidemiologist at the University of Michigan School of Public Health.

In the call for more research on the interactions between the menstrual cycle and women's overall health, Harlow notes inconclusive evidence that the timing of breast-cancer surgery during the menstrual cycle influences a woman's chances of survival. A 1991 report in the medical journal *Lancet* found that women with node-positive premenopausal breast cancer who had surgery after ovulation, when progesterone is present, had up to 30 percent better survival rates than similar women who had surgery before ovulation, when estrogen levels are highest and progesterone is largely absent.

Some limited information is available on factors that could affect the menstrual cycle, such as stress, diet, and exposure to common environmental chemicals. However the call for more research in these areas has been sounded.

Fertility and pregnancy
The monthly cycle of fertility and bleeding can be changed by a variety of factors, the most obvious of

which are pregnancy and menopause. Hormone-based birth-control methods such as the Pill also alter the cycle significantly. The following sections describe what changes in your cycle when you're on the Pill, pregnant, or menopausal.

Your cycle during pregnancy or on the Pill

At ovulation, which occurs around the midpoint of your cycle, an egg is released and travels from the ovary through the Fallopian tube to the uterus. If the egg meets a sperm on the way, fertilization can occur. If fertilization is going to happen during a cycle, it tends to occur within 24 hours of ovulation, while the egg is still in the Fallopian tube.

Fertilization changes the hormonal rhythms that would normally result in a period. Progesterone, which normally is highest during the second half of the cycle, rises dramatically during pregnancy—to nearly 10 times its normal peak luteal phase levels—to help support a new life.

Because progesterone is actually secreted from the used-up egg sac, how can so much of it be produced during pregnancy? The answer is that the placenta takes over the job of pumping out the hormone. During pregnancy, the placenta also becomes the female body's major source of estrogen.

When women use oral contraceptives that contain synthetic estrogen and progestin, they do not ovulate. The high levels of estrogen and progestin contained in birth control pills prevent the secretion of FSH and LH via negative feedback. Without FSH and LH, ovulation will not occur. The high levels of hormones present during pregnancy have the same effect on FSH and LH, which is why ovulation does not occur during pregnancy either.

Your cycle leading up to and during menopause

As menopause approaches, women may have cycles during which their sex-hormone levels are inconsistent, and they may not ovulate. The timing of periods may become irregular as well. Consider Joanie's experience:

JOANIE'S STORY

My experiences with perimenopause started two and a half years ago when I had an extra period and since Mom had always told me that blood appearing any time besides the monthly period was probably a sign of cancer, I panicked and went straight to the emergency room. Nobody seemed alarmed, and I had my blood pressure taken, and was given a pelvic exam. Everything seemed to be normal, and the doctor told me not to worry about it. However, I was told that since I was only 44, I couldn't be experiencing perimenopause. How wrong she was.

I had regular periods for at least two years after that, but at least three times a year, I was plagued with the lower back ache. Oh yes, and then there is the bloating that appears way before my period does. Now that I'm 47, the periods are not occurring every month, and I'm having some mild hot flashes. The hot flashes usually happen during the night. They don't keep me awake. I just get up wash my face, drink a big glass of water and go back to bed.

Right now, I'm doing all right most of the time. I have also learned from my doctor and from people on (a) menopause (mailing) list that spotting is okay during perimenopause. You can bet that I told my mom all about that.

During perimenopause and up through menopause, what causes changes in the frequency and timing of periods? In part, it's an issue of supply and demand.

The number of follicles in the ovary, in which eggs are produced, is limited, and when they are depleted, they are not replaced by new ones. These follicles also produce estrogen. So the depletion of follicles as a woman gets older means a concurrent reduction in the amount of estrogen produced by the ovaries. Without sufficient estrogen secretion, the maturation and release of an egg can't occur—

Timesaver
Check the Internet for resources on fertility planning and calendar-keeping. You can even find software for these purposes.

a situation that holds up other processes (namely the production of progesterone) that would otherwise lead to monthly menstruation. Indeed, if estrogen isn't stimulating the buildup of the endometrium, there is no excess uterine lining to be shed during a menstrual period.

FSH levels typically rise around menopause, as a woman's body tries to spur estrogen production, responding indirectly to a reduced level of the hormone. For similar reasons, levels of LH and another hormone, GnRH, typically shoot up to 3 or 4 times their premenopausal values in women older than 60.

GnRH is short for *gonadotropin-releasing hormone,* a neurohormone that's also called *luteinizing hormone-releasing hormone (LHRH).* This hormone stimulates synthesis and release of LH and FSH from the pituitary gland.

Once a hormone is produced, how does it actually have an effect on the body? After all, hormones are produced from their various glands and are then carried in the bloodstream bathing all parts of the body equally. Why then does the uterus bleed when exposed to estrogen while the heart does not?

In order to fully understand how your body reacts to hormones, the concept of hormone receptors needs to be explained. Hormone receptors are located on the surface of the body's cells. They are the crucial link that allows a cell to recognize a hormone. Once a receptor recognizes the appropriate hormone, the free hormone attaches to it, and this sets off a series of chemical reactions inside the cell. It is these reactions that cause the body to show the effects of the hormone. Different cells have different receptors. Cells that lack the appropriate receptor will not react to the hormone. A hormone is similar to a key. Just like a key will only open certain doors, hormones will only fit into their appropriate receptors. Some hormones function like master keys—the type of key that will open many doors in a particular building. These hormones have effects on many of the body's locked doors. Other hormones are very specific, only affecting a limited number of cells in the body. This concept of hormone receptors is important in understanding a whole new class of medications that have recently become available in treating menopause. We will discuss this in a later chapter.

A month in the life of your menstrual cycle

If you haven't yet entered menopause but are concerned with perimenopause, or if you're just curious, keep a calendar of your menstruation patterns and possible ovulation patterns. This calendar can be an interesting exercise, as well as a potentially valuable resource for you and your doctor.

Whether or not you chart your ovulation patterns, keeping a chart of all bleeding is important for your health. The bleeding patterns or lack of pattern become important information that can help your doctor diagnose abnormal conditions. At the very least, it can help to give you insight into what is happening to your body on a hormonal level. All women should keep some kind of a menstrual diary. It can be as simple as putting a small dot on your personal calendar next to the first day of bleeding.

You can borrow a few tips from the practice of fertility planning and use a chart like the following one.

Note!
Tracking Your
Cycles—Weekly
Calendar.

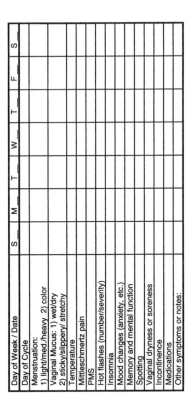

Day of Week / Date	S__	M__	T__	W__	T__	F__	S__
Day of Cycle							
Menstruation: 1) light/med./heavy 2) color							
Vaginal Mucus: 1) wet/dry 2) sticky/slippery/ stretchy							
Temperature							
Mittleschmertz pain							
PMS							
Hot flashes (number/severity)							
Insomnia							
Mood changes (anxiety, etc.)							
Memory and mental function							
Spotting							
Vaginal dryness or soreness							
Incontinence							
Medications							
Other symptoms or notes:							

At least four things can help you tentatively track ovulation:

- Basal body temperature
- Changes in cervical mucus
- Ovulation pain (mittleschmertz)
- Days since the onset of the last period (in very regular women)

Taking your temperature every morning before you get out of bed can give you a good approximation of your basal body temperature and its fluctuations. In the day or hours before ovulation (which generally occurs on day 14 of your monthly cycle), your body temperature sometimes drops, and your

CALENDARS ON THE INTERNET

Menopausal calendars

Thrive Online:
http://thriveonline.com/health/menopause/tools/worksheet.
calendar.html

MENOPAUS mailing list links:
http://www.howdyneighbor.com/menopaus/MenoLinks.htm

Menstrual or fertility planning calendars

Unipath:
http://www.unipath.com/cons004a.htm

Parents' Place:
http://www.pregnancycalendar.com/

Fertility UK
http://www.fertilityuk.org/nfps25.html#indicatorsoffertilityslug

**Downloadable menstrual or fertility planning software &
tools (for purchase, but often with trial period)**

Cyclic:
http://www.queendom.com/cyclic.html

Conceive Fertility Planner(tm)
http://www.wie.com/cfp/

Family of the Americas: Charting Coach:
http://www.familyplanning.net/avoiding.pregnancy.html

Unipath
http://www.unipath.com/cons004a.htm

WombMoon Calendar:
http://www.yoni.com/wombmoon/wmcalinfo.shtml

temperatures are likely to be higher for several days immediately following ovulation. Some women, however, don't have temperatures that correlate well with the times when they're actually fertile, so be advised in case you get funny numbers. Basal-temperature tracking may work best, by the way, when you have no significant disruptions in your health or sleep patterns.

Women who ovulate usually experience some change in their vaginal mucus over the course of the month. A general feeling of wetness or dryness should be noted. Using fingers or a tissue at the opening of the vagina, note whether there seems to be mucus, and whether its seems to be slippery, stretchy, moist, sticky, or some combination. The qualities of mucus play a role in how receptive the vaginal environment is to sperm, encouraging transport into the body during fertile times and discouraging it at others.

A cloudy, sticky mucus with whitish or yellowish color signals that an egg is near release. Just before you ovulate, the mucus becomes more clear and stretchy, not unlike raw egg white. One of the functions of this mucus is thought to be the encouragement of sperm motility.

When gauged by the changing quality of vaginal mucus, ovulation generally occurs a day before or after the last day when you notice a relatively large amount of *slippery* mucus. Obviously, if you are using this method to track ovulation, you must have become familiar with the changes in mucus consistency that are normal for you over the course of several months. These changes are, after all, subjectively determined (slippery, stretchy, sticky, and so on). Bear in mind that douching and yeast or other vaginal infections can alter the consistency of your mucus.

You can also record any other symptoms that you notice during the month that may be related to ovulation or menstruation, such as slight pain or a tug at one of the ovaries. This sensation, known as *mittelschmertz,* may be related to the release of an egg or the events that accompany that release. Some women report feeling heaviness or swelling in their abdomens around the time of ovulation. Record as well any PMS symptoms, cravings, libido changes, or weight fluctuations, if you like.

Watch Out!
The type of tracking explained in this section is not intended to be used for contraceptive planning, so don't rely on it for that purpose! There are no hard-and-fast rules about when a woman will definitely ovulate, particularly when her cycles may already be disrupted during perimenopause.

Libido may increase at around the time of ovulation, and food cravings can occur at different times of the month, particularly just before menstruation. Observe what your craving is for: chocolate, salty and greasy food, meat, or something else. Then see whether a pattern exists.

There is debate about what particular cravings mean, if anything—does a meat craving mean you need iron and protein, or does wanting chocolate mean you need magnesium? Some researchers think women may crave particular foods for their influence on brain chemistry. Most carbohydrates, and other foods that contain the amino acid tryptophan, can increase brain serotonin levels, providing a calming effect. Chocolate, the most-craved food, contains caffeine, theobromine, and the neurotransmitter precursors phenyalanine and tyrosine. However, research seems to indicate that it's the *sensory* properties of the food craved that constitute the craving, rather than the nutrients the food contains.

Women have been found to eat from 90 to 500 calories more per day, and to consume more carbohydrate, protein, fat, vitamin D, riboflavin, potassium, phosphorus, and magnesium during the luteal phase of their menstrual cycle than in their follicular phase. Some researchers posit that the body's increased heat production may be associated with these higher intakes.

Also record the days when you actually have your period. You may want to note the general color, amount, and clottiness of the blood. What you find out about the general characteristics of your cycle may help both you and your doctor decide how to proceed with any difficulties that you're experiencing.

Just the facts

- The first day of menstruation is day 1 of the menstrual cycle, which typically runs 26 to 28 days, with ovulation often occurring near day 14.

- A finite number of ovarian follicles produce estrogen, and as they are depleted over time and ovulatory cycles, the rate of estrogen production drops, leading to menopause.

- The three major types of estrogen produced by the body, in order of strength, are estradiol, estrone, and estriol.

GET THE SCOOP ON...
Hormonal changes ▪ Infertility, PMS, and
menopause ▪ The impact of stress ▪ Factors that
affect the menopausal experience ▪ Common
conditions in perimenopause and menopause

What Can Go Wrong

Chapter 5

How far reaching are perimenopause and menopause problems? Quite. One study found that as many as 20 percent of women experience difficulty on a day-to-day basis. The healthy body has a remarkable capability to repair itself, balance systems that fall out of sync, and restore order from chaos. But when the normal hormonal balance that a woman has become accustomed to for the bulk of her adult life starts to run haywire as is seen in problematic perimenopause, the disruption tends to affect many facets of a woman's life.

This chapter guides you through the hormonal changes that herald menopause and detail how they're connected to some of the difficulties that women may encounter along the way.

Decline and fall of the hormone empire

The strength and balance of hormones help account for the vibrancy of youth and healthy adulthood. The phenomenal development of the body during gestation, infancy, childhood, and adolescence relies on powerful hormonal triggers. At the onset of puberty, a sharp rise occurs in the release of growth hormone and gonadotropic hormones (FSH and LH) from the anterior pituitary, which in the female stimulates estrogen in the ovaries. The release of estrogens prompts the development of the feminine figure, with larger breasts and wider hips, and also initiates the menstrual cycle and fertility. Androgens, the so-called male hormones, also play a role, spurring the growth of pubic and axillary (underarm) hair.

But with age and illness comes slowing in the production of many hormones—not just the sex hormones. As you enter your 30s, the amount of growth hormone that your body produces drops about 14 percent each decade, meaning that by the typical retirement age, the output of HGH (human growth hormone) can be half the levels of early adulthood.

The figure on the next page shows how levels of the female sex hormones estradiol and progesterone decline with perimenopause and menopause.

After menopause reduces the output of your female sex hormones, your body's response to that reduction stabilizes. But the road to menopause is not always smooth. Declining hormone levels, hormonal imbalances, and complications from diet, disease, and other factors set up the potential for problems associated with menopause years ahead of time.

What happens when hormone levels change?

Gradual hormonal decline can result in menopausal symptoms that don't arrive all at once, but creep up on you instead. Things just aren't as they used to be.

Moneysaver
Some alternative-medicine practitioners advocate expensive human-growth-hormone injections to combat aging. Certain amino acids (such as arginine, ornithine, glutamine, and lysine) are thought to stimulate growth-hormone production. But a cost-free way to support growth hormone in your body is to get regular exercise and a good night's sleep.

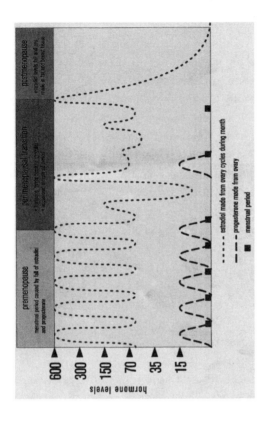

← Note!
Although levels of estrogen, progesterone, and other hormones decrease at menopause, levels of other hormones, such as FSH and LH, increase. FSH and LH stimulate sex-hormone production and reflect the body's attempt to boost sex-hormone levels.

Your periods, levels of energy, weight, skin tone, and emotional stability may shift slightly over several years, and you can be tempted to attribute them to the simple fact of aging. It may not be until (and unless) symptoms become severe that you even *think* to associate them with menopause. But if you question your symptoms with menopause in mind right off the bat, you have a fighting chance of addressing them and improving your pre-menopausal years—perhaps even maintaining your fertility longer and easing your transition through menopause when it finally arrives.

If you know in advance that changes in the body may be menopause-related, you're in a position to request hormone-level testing from your doctor. The results of such testing can help you consider what, if any, steps to take—from addressing nutrition and stress issues in your life to, possibly, initiating hormone-replacement therapy. In early, subtle cases of hormone change, adding specifically supportive foods and nutrients to your diet may ameliorate problems and make a dramatic change in your vitality (see Chapter 10 for more details on nutrition and menopause).

In the years before menopause, your levels of estrogen and progesterone are declining but not always in sync. A decline in estrogen production can mean that during a particular cycle, your ovarian follicles may not mature and release an egg properly or on time, resulting in a lack of progesterone production. (See Chapter 4 for information on how this domino effect occurs).

In such a cycle, although inadequate *estrogen* production may be the root of the problem, some physicians believe that the resulting deficiency in *progesterone* can lead a woman to experience symptoms of *hormonal imbalance*—that is, too much estrogen in relation to progesterone. These symptoms include irritability, headaches, bloating, and other effects that are commonly lumped together under the term *premenstrual syndrome (PMS)*.

Bright Idea
Check out Chapter 13 for information about the multitude of ways that you can use herbs to address typical menopause discomforts. Some herbs have a reputation for assisting in balancing hormones.

Perimenopause and menopause— Just what is happening to me?

Once the normal fluctuations that occur in the menstrual cycle are understood, it becomes easier to understand exactly what the changes are that occur with the onset of perimenopause and how the hormonal fluctuations that occur result in the changes women experience.

When does the perimenopausal transition start? One easily identified event is the point in time that menstrual irregularities begin. In American women this occurs at 47.5 years of age. We know from more sophisticated hormonal studies that prior to the onset of irregular periods, there are more subtle changes that can be detected. It is this knowledge that is responsible for the increased awareness of early perimenopausal changes (and may even be the reason you are reading this book in the first place). The very earliest changes can start to occur at the average age of 35. This is when a statistical decrease of fertility is seen, although many women still have excellent fertility at this time. (Remember that this is just an average age based on statistical analysis of a large number of women and doesn't necessarily reflect any one individual person. There are wide fluctuations in age of onset of peri-menopause and menopause as well as large varia-tions in fertility.)

Unofficially...
If the eggs could remain "ageless" and never decrease their activity or their number, menopause and all its symptoms wouldn't happen. Women would just keep on menstruating and conceiving, month after month and year after year.

Changes during early perimenopause

The real reason that menopause occurs in the first place is that the eggs become older and less respon-sive to stimulating hormones (FSH and LH). The pituitary gland is forced to produce increasing levels of FSH in an attempt to induce a susceptible follicle to ovulate. As ever greater levels of FSH are produced several hormonal changes begin to occur in regularly ovulating women. (Remember, this is still the early phase when a missed ovulation has not yet occurred.)

- The follicles respond to the increased FSH stimulus, and they produce elevated levels of estradiol. During this phase there is a very prominent amount of clear cervical mucus at

Watch Out!
Menopause may
be hastened and
perimenopause
provoked or
exacerbated by
serious bodily
stressors, such as
smoking,
chemotherapy,
disease, or sim-
ply a stressful
lifestyle.

the time of ovulation. Some women experience heavier periods at this early phase.

- The follicular phase (first half of the menstrual cycle) becomes shorter resulting in a progressively shorter total menstrual cycle length.

- There is a greater tendency to have double ovulations (due to increased FSH) which is why fraternal twinning is more common as women age.

- Fertility may start to decline as evidenced by a longer time to successful conception and a greater tendency to miscarry.

Some fertility specialists will measure hormone levels during the early part of the menstrual cycle in order to get a handle on a woman's reproductive capacity. Blood tests measuring levels of FSH and estradiol are taken on the second or third day of the menstrual cycle. During this early part of the cycle the levels should normally be low. In women with decreased fertility potential these levels tend to be elevated, a reflection of the ovarian follicles' resistance to FSH. As the follicles become less responsive to FSH, the pituitary is forced to produce ever higher amounts of the hormone in an attempt to produce an ovulation. The follicles themselves, during this early phase, respond to the increased FSH hormone by producing higher estradiol levels. Fertility specialists see the elevated levels as an indication that special procedures such as in vitro fertilization may not be successful. Bear in mind that many women with levels in this range can still conceive spontaneously since there is a marked variation in these levels from cycle to cycle and from woman to woman. These tests should be used as a guide, as a way to get a handle on things.

Changes during late perimenopause

As the ovarian follicles become increasingly less responsive to FSH, menstrual irregularities increase. The ovarian follicles start to "burn out" and the production of estradiol declines. Sometimes ovulation doesn't even occur, despite the added push of elevated FSH. These unresponsive eggs are too "pooped to pop," like the unpopped kernels of corn at the bottom of a microwaved bag of popcorn. During this late perimenopausal phase several different symptoms start to show up:

- Periods become increasingly unpredictable and irregular, sometimes with long intervals of time between bleeding (*amenorrhea,* the medical term for prolonged absence of periods). These intervals will often be followed by a series of regular ovulatory cycles.

- It is not unusual for women to start to experience hot flashes and night sweats during the phases of amenorrhea. These symptoms are the result of low estrogen levels.

- As regular ovulatory cycles become interspersed with the phases of amenorrhea, the hot flashes disappear, evidence of increased estradiol becomes apparent (such as the reappearance of clear cervical mucus), and the body feels like it did before.

- Menstrual periods will often become lighter and shorter. Occasional heavy periods and spotting in between periods is not unusual either. Menstrual irregularities will be discussed in detail later in this chapter.

- Some women experience vaginal dryness and pain during intercourse as a result of lowered estradiol levels.

■ It is not unusual for the testosterone levels to
rise at this time. As FSH and LH increase in
their attempt to spur on yet another ovulation,
they also stimulate the rest of the ovarian tissue,
the stroma, where testosterone is produced.
This is further amplified by decreasing levels of
estradiol, which allows a greater amount of free
testosterone to circulate in the body. For most
women this elevated testosterone gives not only
a sense of well-being and increased energy, but
also gives a boost to sexual desire (libido).

■ The hormonal fluctuations of this phase of
perimenopause often cause emotional upheaval
for many women. The roller-coaster hormonal
highs and lows can have major emotional effects
on some women.

The late perimenopausal phase by the very
nature of a lack of order that was seen before these
changes started is a hormonal "mixed bag."
Hormone testing during this phase must be interpreted with the individual woman's situation in
mind at that particular point in time. Thus, drawing
blood levels of FSH and estradiol at a time when hot
flashes are prominent and amenorrhea is present,
will usually yield levels consistent with menopause.
In this situation FSH will be markedly elevated and
estradiol will be low. If the same blood tests are then
drawn two or three months later when ovulatory
cycles have resumed, one might see a picture consistent with that of a younger woman. Blood tests will
offer an objective measurement that can sometimes
be helpful, but they must always be interpreted with
the events around which they are drawn.

During a routine gynecologic exam evidence of
estradiol presence or absence can many times be

detected. Cervical mucus, when present, is very obvious. The vagina is very sensitive to the effects of estradiol. When estradiol levels are high, the vagina has a thick, lush appearance; when absent, it becomes thinned out and shiny. This effect can be seen on the routine PAP smear. A "maturity index" can be requested at the time a PAP smear is taken. The cytologist in the lab then makes an assessment of the level of estrogen effect on the vaginal cells. Because the vagina is so sensitive to estrogen, these effects can be readily seen. Keep in mind that this is a qualitative reading, which means it only gives a rough assessment, but one that may be helpful to you nonetheless.

Changes during menopause
Menopause is the true end to a woman's reproductive capacity. Natural ovulation will not occur since the eggs have been depleted. The ovarian follicles, the sacs around the eggs that produce estrogen, also become unresponsive to FSH, and estrogen levels drop markedly. From a practical point of view menopause can be said to occur when there have been no menstrual periods for one year.

Hormonal changes that started in the perimenopausal phase intensify during menopause. Not only does FSH increase, but LH now shows an increase as well. Estradiol levels decrease, and estrone becomes the major estrogen in the body.

Hormones are produced from two major sources in the body: the ovary and the adrenal gland.

As mentioned earlier, the ovary produces hormones from the ovarian follicles (estrogen and progesterone) and from the stroma, the tissue surrounding the follicles (testosterone). With

Moneysaver
By keeping a diary or mental log of your symptoms (cervical mucus presence or absence, hot flashes, bleeding patterns, premenstrual symptoms) you can get a reasonable idea of where you stand hormonally with respect to perimenopause.

decreasing follicular responsiveness to FSH and LH, the ovarian stroma becomes stimulated by these hormones. The production of testosterone can increase after menopause. As menopause progresses over years this testosterone production decreases as well.

The adrenal contribution becomes relatively more prominent during menopause as estradiol decreases. Androgens from the adrenal gland diminish slowly with age but are not affected specifically by menopausal changes the way ovarian hormones are. These androgens are converted to estrone in "peripheral tissue" such as the fat, skin, and muscle. Heavier women have more estrone than thin women.

Here are a few interesting hormonal concepts regarding menopause:

- Most tissues in the body have estrogen receptors. The decline in total estrogen during menopause has far reaching effects that become more prominent over time. For example, effects are seen in the vagina and urinary bladder as well as in the bones, brain, and liver. We know for example that cholesterol production is affected and less favorable cholesterol increases while "good" cholesterol decreases.

- Estrone effects can be significant in certain women. Since ovulation doesn't occur in menopause, progesterone is not produced. This can result in estrogen excess, that is estrogen that is not balanced by progesterone. The endometrium, the lining of the uterus can become overstimulated by estrogen resulting in endometrial hyperplasia, which is an abnormal response of the lining to excessive hormones.

This condition can progress to endometrial carcinoma (cancer of the lining of the uterus). It is important that women who have bleeding during menopause contact their physicians so they can be properly evaluated for this condition.

- Hair growth on the chin and face may increase during menopause due to the relative increase in the proportion of androgens during menopause.

Although physicians largely agree that hormonal imbalances underlie menopause-related complaints, there is less general certainty about which hormones cause what positive and negative effects—a testament to the intricacy of the balance that must be maintained for health and comfort.

The body's quest for balance

An intricate network of feedback systems regulates the production and use of hormones, neurotransmitters (brain chemicals that regulate body functions), and other bodily messengers with exquisite precision. Your body is always seeking balance through a phenomenon known as *homeostasis*—a fact that is both a great strength and a great weakness. When one aspect of the feedback loop changes, another changes as well, to compensate. The decline of estrogen production by the ovaries during perimenopause and menopause, for example, doesn't mean the end of estrogen for the female body. Instead, the body increasingly relies upon usable estrogen produced elsewhere, such as in fat cells and the adrenal glands.

A significant amount of estrogen in the form of estrone can be produced in the fat cells of the body. The greater the amount of fat, the greater the estrone production. Estrone is a weaker estrogen than estradiol but if enough of it is produced, the effects can be significant. This is the reason obese women usually have fewer hot flashes than women of normal body weight. They tend to have less wrinkled skin, stronger bones, and less vaginal thinning. They also have a greater risk of endometrial cancer due to higher unbalanced estrogen levels.

But your body's constant search for balance can make it difficult to discover the proper treatment, should problems arise. Adding a little extra amount of one substance may send unanticipated signals to your body to increase levels of another substance to maintain homeostasis. That intricate network of feedback systems is still hard at work. The job of handling menopause difficulties requires a delicate touch.

Unofficially...
Some doctors say that hormone-replacement therapy with natural progesterone and estrogen may be better tolerated than conventional replacement therapy. They say natural progesterone, in particular, doesn't produce the same side effects as progestins and ameliorates the symptoms for which progestins are blamed. But the topic is still being hotly debated.

In conventional gynecology, estrogen is often thought of as being "the happy hormone" because of its buoyant effects on mood and well-being. It has, therefore, gained a good reputation in hormone-replacement therapy, although individual women respond to it in different ways, and more than a few have difficulty adjusting to it. The progestins that are frequently given as supplements at the same time, however, may not be tolerated as well; in fact, they are frequently blamed for the irritability and other symptoms of PMS. Part 3 of this book provides more information about this dilemma.

Early warning: perimenopause

Instead of a gracefully orchestrated finale to their fertile years, some women experience a clumsy cacophony of hormonal signals for several years, beginning as early as the 30s, as the body tries to sort out where it wants to be, hormonally speaking.

Out-of-step levels of any of the sex hormones generate other problems in the body. These problems manifest themselves as the symptoms of perimenopause—that is, menopausal symptoms that occur before the onset of true menopause.

From contraception to perimenopause?

Birth-control pills are, in effect, a form of hormone-replacement therapy, and much as hormone-replacement therapy can reduce or eliminate menopause-related problems, the Pill can relieve or mask perimenopausal problems.

Each pill provides a steady stream of hormones (usually, estrogen and a progestin), thus eliminating the normal rise and fall of the natural hormones in the body. The high levels of synthetic hormones force FSH and LH to plummet. This inhibits ovulation and stops the ovaries from producing hormones. During the week that you take placebo pills (or no pill at all), your body recognizes that its daily supply of hormones has stopped, allowing menstruation to occur. This is why, if you've used birth-control pills for years and then switch to another, nonhormonal form of birth control, you may suddenly find yourself in the midst of perimenopause, experiencing irregular periods, PMS, and other difficulties.

The Pill is not believed to cause a woman to go into perimenopause, but it may mask the changes she would be experiencing during her late 30s or early 40s if she was not on the medication. By the same token, very low dose birth-control pills can now be used as treatment for perimenopausal symptoms in those women who desire contraception, are nonsmokers, and are having annoying symptoms during this transition.

Some people claim that this phenomenon is biological evidence that "it's not nice to fool Mother Nature," arguing that the continued use of birth-control pills may lead to imbalances in the body's *own* production and use of hormones. After all, these people say, birth-control pills don't just prevent pregnancy, but also prevent the natural fertility cycle, beginning with ovulation itself. But while the Pill does prevent ovulation, current scientific literature suggests it does not permanently affect fertility (however, the return of fertility may be temporarily delayed).

But the Pill has long been touted as a preventive for pregnancy and disease and as a treatment for some conditions (see Part 3 of this book). Birth-control pills are frequently prescribed as treatment for irregular periods, painful periods (dysmenorrhea), effects of excessive androgen production (such as acne and excessive body hair growth), and heavy menstrual flow. Recent studies have shown that the Pill can decrease the incidence of ovarian cancer by 60 percent if used for at least 6 years. Among the more unusual theories in support of birth-control pills is the argument that too many ovulations in a woman's lifetime (once a month) are in themselves unnatural, hastening menopause by depleting the number of egg-containing follicles in a woman's ovaries. That is to say, in the natural course of things *without* some kind of birth control, frequent pregnancies could be expected, which would result in fewer lifetime ovulations, as shown in Table 5.1.

TABLE 5.1: PREGNANCY'S IMPACT ON LIFETIME OVULATION

Years of Fertility (35)	Lifetime Ovulations
With 0 pregnancies	420
With 10 pregnancies	270

Infertility and perimenopause

Infertility can be symptomatic of perimenopause-related hormonal imbalance, especially when childbearing is delayed as it has been increasingly over the last several decades. How widespread is infertility? It may be even more pronounced in our culture than statistics suggest because, unless a couple is actively trying to produce a child, infertility may not be investigated or detected. One of every 6 to 10 couples experiences infertility, and about 60 percent of the time, the problem involves the female. Following are some of the reasons for infertility:

- Disturbances in the ovulatory cycle

- Hormonal imbalances such as luteal phase deficiency

- Endometriosis

- Pelvic infection, such as pelvic inflammatory disease

- Polycystic Ovarian Syndrome (PCO)

- Immune-system problems

- Structural abnormalities of the uterus (fibroids, polyps, as well as congenital defects such as, an abnormally shaped uterus which 2 percent of women are born with)

- Other genetic or acquired disorders

← **Note!**
A woman who is fertile for 35 years and has 10 pregnancies experiences a reduction of more than 35 percent in the number of lifetime ovulations, compared with a woman who is never pregnant, assuming that she has had no nonovulatory cycles outside of pregnancy and lactation. (Numbers cited in table are estimates).

When age alone is a factor in decreasing fer-tility, one well-known study looked at fertility rates among Hutterite women in a community in which contraception was not used. The percentage of no further pregnancies as related to age is as follows:

- By age 34: 11 percent
- By age 39: 33 percent
- By age 44: 87 percent

Infertility is not the only problem associated with aging: Miscarriage also becomes increasingly more common as women age. The most important factor causing this increased incidence of miscarriage is the genetic imbalances that result from "older" eggs. This is why Down's syndrome, which is just one potential chromosomal abnormality, increases with increasing maternal age. Nature recognizes most of these genetic abnormalities as being incompatible with life, and miscarriage occurs. Another less common cause for miscarriage in older women is a hormonal imbalance called luteal phase defect. This is the result of decreased progesterone levels that are inadequate to maintain the pregnancy in the uterus. Sometimes miscarriage occurs because of irregularities in the inner surface of the uterus due to endometrial polyps and fibroids, both of which are more common in women in the early perimenopausal years.

How much more frequent is miscarriage in older women? Miscarriage occurs in 12 percent of women age 20 but jumps to 26 percent in women age 40—and increases even more dramatically after the age of 40. In vitro fertilization technology using an ovum donation is one option for fertility in women whose low fertility is due to the perimenopausal and even the menopausal process. Success rates with this technology can be excellent.

PMS and perimenopause

More than half of the women in the United States may experience premenstrual syndrome (PMS) at some time during their fertile years, including symptoms as wide ranging as the following:

- Aches and pains
- Acne and other skin problems
- Aggressiveness
- Alcohol intolerance
- Anxiety
- Asthma
- Back pain
- Bloating
- Blood-pressure and heart-rate abnormalities
- Breast tenderness and swelling
- Bruising
- Clumsiness
- Cramps
- Cravings (sweets, chocolate, salty or fatty foods, and/or protein)
- Depression
- Fainting
- Fatigue
- Headache
- Hemorrhoidal or herpes flare-ups
- Insomnia
- Irritability
- Lethargy

Watch Out!
Smoking has an adverse effect on fertility during the peri-menopausal years. Smoking has been shown to speed up the onset of menopause by 1.5 years.

Watch Out!
See your physician about any serious symptoms. Underlying disorders may require prompt treatment to prevent the development of disease.

- Mood swings
- Nausea
- Seizures
- Sinus problems
- Sore throat
- Urination difficulty
- Vision abnormalities

Some typical PMS symptoms can be tied together. An interesting study published in the *Journal of Affective Disorders* in 1995 noted the incidence of food cravings and depression in women during various phases of their menstrual cycle. In each phase, the severity of the food craving turned out to be very strongly related to the severity of depression that the women reported. Researchers at the University of Leeds in England found that the more they craved food, the less happiness women reported in their relationships. The study also found some correlation between that effect and ongoing stress. Food cravings also occurred without depression and tended to be reported most just before the period began (no surprise there).

Premenstrual symptoms can range from the slightly uncomfortable to the disabling. Although many women find that their difficulties begin a few days before menstruation and end when menstruation begins, premenstrual symptoms can—and frequently do—occur elsewhere in the cycle. Some women's discomfort stretches from around the time of ovulation through the beginning of the period. Still others develop difficulties during the postperiod phase. In every case, the symptoms indicate that the body is out of balance.

Bright Idea
Some food cravings may be your body's way of asking for the right raw material from which to make the hormones and neurotransmitters that it needs for your emotional balance. See Chapter 10 for information on what cravings can mean that you're *really* low on.

Similarly, women differ in their lifelong experience of PMS. Some women experience PMS from the onset of their periods; others, only during times of particular stress. Many women's PMS symptoms increase in severity as they get closer to menopause, however; so for them, premenstrual syndrome can't be separated from perimenopause.

From frustration to flushing

Although women often experience PMS and infertility at around the time of natural menopause, other difficulties that are characteristic of the soon-to-come climacteric occur in younger women who are undergoing perimenopause. The symptoms include, but aren't limited to, the typical hot flashes, vaginal dryness, urinary difficulties and infections, and reduced libido. Any menopausal symptoms can also occur during perimenopause, which is part of the same continuum.

If you're having a hot flash, you should know not just what you're feeling and how to treat it, but also the cause—why you're uncomfortable in the first place. Simply put, hot flashes are caused by hormonal changes occurring in your body. Your body periodically perceives a relative decrease in estrogen levels, which causes your FSH levels to increase. This rise in FSH is believed to bring about the physical sensation of the "hot flash."

The importance of learning the "why" of your physical symptoms applies to *any* ailment that you encounter. By taking a close look at where your body isn't finding balance, you'll be better able to find the root of the dissynchrony and remedy the real problem, and perhaps save yourself from other problems that can be attributed to the same cause.

Watch Out!
As many as three out of every five women experience cramps. Although they are often part of PMS, cramps can also indicate an underlying disease, such as endometriosis.

Conditions and symptoms that can occur or become more pronounced during both perimenopause and menopause include the following:

- Dysmenorrhea (cramps; painful menstruation).

- Amenorrhea (abnormally absent or suppressed menstruation).

- PMS (variety of cyclical discomforts).

- Dysfunctional uterine bleeding (irregular periods, including spotting).

- Endometrial hyperplasia (overgrowth of endometrial glands resulting from overstimulation of the uterine lining, usually due to an excess of estrogen and a relative deficiency of progesterone).

- Endometriosis (growth of uterine-lining tissue in other pelvic areas).

- Fibroids (fibrous growths or benign tumors in the uterus). Also known as myomas, fibroids are very common in women (30 percent have them). They often grow during perimenopause and, along with hormonal imbalances, are responsible for many bleeding abnormalities that occur during this time.

- Ovarian cysts and polycystic ovarian syndrome (cysts in the ovaries arising from hormonal disruption and associated with irregular periods).

- Ovarian cancer. The incidence increases after age 40. It appears to be an age-related phenomenon rather than a direct response to menopause.

- Vaginal and urinary infections. The vagina and bladder are very sensitive to estrogen. They become less resistant to bacteria as thinning occurs.

- Vaginal dryness and thinning, leading to pain during intercourse and making infection more likely.

- Breast cancer. The incidence increases after age 40.

- Hot flashes. The result of lower estrogen and higher FSH levels.

- Migraine headaches. Sometimes headaches are exacerbated by hormonal shifts.

- Osteoporosis. This is the result of aging and lowered estrogen levels.

- Hair thinning and loss. These are the effects of aging, genetic predisposition, and relative androgen excess.

- Depression and moodiness, caused by hormonal fluctuations.

- Insomnia, possibly due to interrupted sleep resulting from night sweats.

- Night sweats—hot flashes occurring at night.

- Menorrhagia—the regular, cyclic bleeding that is heavier than usual.

- Metrorrhagia—bleeding that occurs at other than the normal time for a woman's menstrual period.

- Menometrorrhagia—a combination of heavy menstrual flow with abnormal bleeding between periods.

Parts 3 and 4 of this book deal in detail with these conditions and their treatments.

What affects perimenopause and menopause?

The question could just as easily be "what *doesn't* affect perimenopause and menopause?" Although both terms are used to describe complaints of a gynecological nature, the effects and causes involve the entire woman. Following are some of the major contributors to the onset of perimenopause and menopause:

- Genetic predisposition
- Radiation therapy if directed to the pelvis
- Presence of disease
- Certain environmental toxins or harsh medications such as some chemotherapy agents if given during the late reproductive life
- Smoking, which hastens the onset of menopause by an average of 1.5 years.

Bright Idea
See Chapter 9 for the lowdown about what scientists are learning about the effect of environmental toxins on hormone levels.

Your background and perimenopause

Like it or not, you're stuck with your relatives, including those who came before you and whose genetic material you've inherited. Ask about your family history. If close female relatives typically reached menopause at a young age, you may be predisposed to do so as well, so you may want to take particular care to bolster your health and support your hormones with that fact in mind. Similarly, find out how late in life women in your family gave birth. The older the mother, the longer her fertility may have lasted—another clue for you about your own situation.

Your age when you first began to menstruate may also play a role. Multiple studies have found no correlation between age at onset of menstruation and age at onset of menopause; other studies hint that these two statistics may go together. But looking at risk factors for such menopause-related issues as osteoporosis, Japanese researchers found that early menopause was associated with low bone-mineral density and that early *menarche* (age at menstrual onset) had a relationship to high bone-mineral density. The role of estrogen in protecting the bones is now well known, and it can be said that (if all other things are equal) early menopause limits lifetime estrogen output, whereas early menarche increases it.

You are what you eat

Inadequate nutrition can set you up for problems during perimenopause and menopause. Some foods, however, may help relieve you of many menopausal symptoms.

A significant number of adult Americans don't get the recommended daily intake of common vitamins and minerals. Emphasis on low-fat and unsafe or fad diets can also seriously curtail the supply of essential fatty acids and protein that your body needs. Perimenopausal problems can be provoked by vitamin or mineral deficiency, and can themselves increase the need for certain nutrients. Unusually heavy periods have the potential to set up iron-deficiency anemia, which is experienced by 10 percent of menstruating women. Chapter 10 describes realistic ways to prevent such deficiencies.

Certain foods may help relieve the symptoms of perimenopause and menopause. At the moment there's a great deal of interest in soy. Japanese women, whose diet typically is very high in soybean-derived foods, experience menopausal problems at a fraction of the rate that American women do. In addition, Asian women who eat a traditional low-fat diet with plentiful soy are reported to have a 4-to-6-times-lower risk of developing breast cancer.

Other foods and herbs contain phytoestrogens, which enhance hormonal activity in the body.

Unofficially...
If you'd like to do further reading, an excellent book on the mind–body aspects of women's health is *Women's Bodies, Women's Wisdom* by Christiane Northrup, M.D. See Appendix C for more suggested reading.

These are useful to support flagging estrogen levels and thus can potentially ease hot flashes, improve the look of the skin, and alleviate some hormone-related mood problems. These foods include soy, pumpkin seeds, and flaxseed oil.

Stress: Real effects in your body

Just as stress is a factor in the development of heart disease and other serious conditions, stress can affect the severity of your perimenopausal symptoms and is itself capable of setting off hormonal imbalance. To understand why, you need to examine again how hormones are created, this time paying attention to the way that stress hormones function.

It all starts with cholesterol. Without enough cholesterol, you can't manufacture the steroid hormones that are needed to support a wide range of functions. From cholesterol, the body makes pregnenolone, which in turn is used to create progesterone. From that compound, the body can make corticosterone and cortisol—two important stress hormones that help regulate energy in the body and participate in the response of your immune system. These hormones also play a primary role in regulating your response to stress. Estrogen production is farther down the chain of steroid development.

The more stress your body encounters, the more your adrenal glands are taxed to produce certain hormones. In evolutionary terms, these hormones are designed to help you respond to danger with supranormal surges of energy (the fight-or-flight response). When a wild animal is at your heels, these hormone surges are a good thing. The hormone surges can be too much, however, when the same response is invoked daily by mundane events such as drinking caffeine, fighting morning traffic, having

Bright Idea
Adding soy-based foods to your diet is one way to increase your phytoestrogen intake. A cup of soybeans is said to have about 300mg of isoflavones, the plant estrogen equivalent of one typically prescribed estrogen tablet.

a doughnut (the overload of sugar stresses your adrenals), and worrying about work deadlines.

The adrenal medulla—the inner part of an adrenal gland—is hard-wired into your nervous system. Here, with the help of corticosteroids, your body changes your heart rate and alters your blood sugar and blood pressure, thereby kicking off or shutting down your stress reactions. The adrenal medulla accomplishes these tasks through the actions of adrenaline (epinephrine) and noradrenaline (norepinephrine).

Imagine your body's normal progression of hormone development. Everything's chugging along as it should be. Cholesterol is turning into pregnenolone, and some of that substance is turning into progesterone, which in turn is getting ready to convert to androstenedione, from which the estrogens (estrone, estriol, and estradiol) will be made. Suddenly, the progesterone that is destined to become estrogen (and perhaps a bit of testosterone) is needed elsewhere, in the corticosterone and cortisol departments. Apparently, some major crisis is under way, and the stress-hormone department is leaning on the buzzer for more resources. The body diverts the progesterone from its intended duty to calm the crisis of the moment. Imbalances occur in the pituitary gland, where feedback mechanisms prevent the proper release of FSH and LH.

If this situation occurs day after day, necessary levels of estrogen, progesterone, and other hormones that maintain your body's ovulation and other functions are not met. A domino effect results. Insufficient estrogen for ovulation means no corpus luteum from the released egg to secrete progesterone during the second half of the

Watch Out!
Estrogen deficiency can play a role in Alzheimer's disease, colo-rectal cancer, and other serious ailments. Anorexics who fail to ovulate have a chronic low estrogen level, which stimulates early menopause and predisposes them to osteoporosis and bone fracture. Do what you can now to keep your hormones balanced and eliminate risk factors.

menstrual cycle, which means that you have insufficient raw material from which to make other hormones.

How can you make sure that you are not overly taxing your adrenals and your ovaries? Cut out stress as much as possible. A little stress is okay—but who really has just a little? Remember that your body treats emotional stress the way that it treats physical stress (and that a bit of exercise can release some of that stored tension). Even if you're coping well, are you doing so in a relaxed, natural manner, or are you on your toes perhaps a little more than necessary? Relaxation lowers your epinephrine and cortisol levels, so do relax; it's good for you!

Following are some typical stressors:

Physical stressors

Illness and injury

Harsh medications

Excessive physical activity

Imbalanced hormones

Extreme heat or cold

Pollution

Smoking

Insufficient sleep

Dietary stressors

Insufficient or imbalanced nutrients

Severe dieting

Junk foods

Caffeine and other stimulants

Mental and emotional stressors

Any negative emotion in quantity

Too much work, not enough play

Unofficially...
Some early physicians attributed a proportion of "female difficulties" to nerves. Today, although much more is known about the causes of hormonal imbalance, medicine is coming back around to a similar idea: that the body's not in balance until the mind and emotions are in sync with it. That idea applies to males as well as to females.

Difficult situations and people

Boredom and lack of engaging activity

Relationship concerns

Although just sitting still may be a great stress reducer, lack of movement or emotion doesn't necessarily provide a complete antidote for stress or a recipe for health. You really need to be involved in some meaningful activity—meditation yoga, tai chi, or Qi Gong are especially helpful in combating stress. Happiness is, in fact, a real contributor to your level of health.

Your symptoms depend on you

Factors that include your ethnicity may make a significant difference in how you experience perimenopause and menopause. A five-year program begun in 1994 set out to identify health factors that change with menopause, to distinguish menopausal shifts from other age-related but nonhormonal changes, and to measure ethnic differences in women's experience of menopause. From the initial screening of 10,000 women, researchers found the following:

- Age-related weight gain can put menopausal women at greater risk for heart disease.

- Menopausal symptoms differ across ethnic groups, as do the treatments used to relieve them. African American women are more likely as a group to have hysterectomies, for example, whereas white women are more likely than other groups to receive hormone-replacement therapy.

The Study of Women's Health Across the Nation (SWAN), funded largely by the National Institute on Aging, tracked 3,700 healthy premenopausal

Watch Out!
Researchers writing for the *Journal of the American Medical Association* have found that daily mental stress (tension, frustration, and sadness) can more than double the risk of certain types of heart disease.

women between the ages of 42 and 52. Other studies found that early menopause *itself* is a risk factor
for later problems. One study, by University of
California—Davis researcher Ellen Gold, found that
women who enter menopause before age 50 experience greater risk of developing heart disease, osteoporosis, and other chronic conditions than do
women who enter menopause later.

Researchers divide symptoms into two categories: those that relate to estrogen and those that
involve other somatic symptoms. Table 5.2 outlines
the difference.

TABLE 5.2: MENOPAUSAL SYMPTOMS

Estrogen-Related Symptoms	Somatic Symptoms
Hot flashes	Difficulty sleeping
Night sweats	Headaches
Vaginal dryness	Racing heart
Urine leakage	Joint, neck, and shoulder stiffness and soreness

Dividing obviously estrogen-related symptoms
from those that may not be estrogen related is an
interesting approach. Researchers who examined
such data found that women in two particular categories experienced more symptoms across the
board:

- Smokers
- Women who reported getting little physical activity

Less-educated women were also found to have
more estrogen-related symptoms and to experience
more heart-racing than other women.

Examining the categories by ethnicity,
researchers found that African Americans have
more estrogen-related symptoms but fewer somatic

Unofficially...
Chinese American
women experi-
ence lower rates
of hot flashes
than women
of other
backgrounds.
Researchers are
curious about
whether this
phenomenon is
linked to diet
and the use
of herbs.

symptoms than other ethnic groups. Hispanic women experienced more urinary leakage and heart-racing than other groups. Asian American women reported the fewest symptoms.

The final results of the SWAN study may be particularly useful in developing treatment guidelines and intervention approaches that take ethnic differences into account. Current understanding of menopausal issues is based largely on the experiences of Caucasian women.

Weight is an interesting issue in the SWAN study as well. Researchers found that increased weight in menopausal Caucasian women was linked with aging rather than with menopausal symptoms. In addition, less-educated women tended to gain more weight, and women who were not using hormone-replacement therapy tended to be heavier than those who were using it.

Weight differences were also ethnically distributed, with Asian women being the leanest, African Americans weighing the most, and Caucasians and Hispanics falling in the center. Obesity was strongly correlated with how well women function on a day-to-day basis as they approach menopause. Table 5.3 describes the variations.

TABLE 5.3: WOMEN'S WEIGHT AND FUNCTIONAL ABILITY

Group	Significant Limitations (Percentage)	Some Limitations (Percentage)
All women	8	12
Asian	2–3	
Caucasian	12–14	
African American	12–14	

Source: SWAN study

← Note! A large part of the SWAN study examined women's ability to perform four daily tasks: walk one block, climb a flight of stairs, bathe and dress, and carry groceries. Women who have significant difficulty in performing these tasks on their own are considered to be functionally limited.

Researchers also found that women who have less education, those who are poor, unemployed, or divorced, and smokers all tend to reach menopause at an earlier age than women who don't fit into those categories.

It's important to remember that for each woman, approaching menopause is an individual affair. We all differ from the average experience. You will do best to listen to your body for cues and to learn about menopause on your own, so that you're very well informed about how to protect your health and communicate with your physician when necessary.

Just the facts

- Menopause is the result of aging of the ovarian follicles.

- Women who enter menopause early have a higher risk of heart disease, osteoporosis, and other chronic diseases.

- Dropping estrogen production can result in cycles during which a woman doesn't ovulate and thus doesn't produce normal progesterone levels, furthering the cycle of imbalance.

- One of every 6 to 10 couples experiences infertility. In females (in whom the problem exists, in most cases), infertility is closely linked with perimenopause.

- Women's difficulties during menopause vary by ethnic background.

GET THE SCOOP ON...
Avoiding osteoporosis ▪ Controversies
in treatments ▪ Hormone-replacement
therapy and breast cancer ▪ Menopause and
Alzheimer's disease

Major Menopause-Linked Health Worries

Chapter 6

A mong every 4 women who are post-menopausal, one is likely to be affected by osteoporosis. Seven of 10 are statistically destined to grapple with heart disease. And over the course of their lives, one in three women will develop cancer of one form or another, including the types that hormone therapy may either help prevent or promote.

The older we get, the greater our chance for developing certain types of disease, and the more important it becomes to preserve our health—by eliminating the risk factors that we can do something about; bolstering our general health through diet and exercise; and taking part in preventative care, including screening to catch disease early in its development (when it can often be stopped).

In this chapter, you learn about major health conditions that are related in some way to menopause and discover whether you're at particular risk of developing them. The chapter starts with

119

the very framework of the female body: the skeleton.

Osteoporosis

Unofficially...
The costs of osteoporosis are estimated to reach $3.8 billion annually, according to a 1984 National Institutes of Health Consensus Development Conference Statement on osteoporosis.

Many women spend plenty of time thinking about their skin, their fat, and sometimes their muscles, but don't spend much time thinking about their bones. We would all be well advised to do so. Two maxims seem to apply to these overlooked stalwarts of our existence: Feed them or need them, and use them or lose them.

Osteoporosis—the gradual loss of bone and reduction of the quality of existing bone—is an indirect killer. As many as 15 million to 20 million people in the United States (men as well as women) are affected by it. There usually are no visible signs of the disease until the woman who has it perhaps falls and breaks a hip or another now-fragile bone. The complications of being laid up with a serious fracture often lead to pain and long-term disability. Nearly 20 percent of hip-fracture patients do not survive for a year.

Even those who have the good health to reach age 90 face sobering risks. Nearly one of every three women and one of every five men will suffer a hip fracture, most of the time because of osteoporosis. According to the National Institutes of Health (in a 1984 Consensus Development Conference Statement on osteoporosis), about 1.3 million fractures each year among those age 45 and older are attributable to osteoarthritis.

Because of the threat of osteoporosis, health authorities recommend that every adult woman should supplement her diet with adequate calcium and vitamin D, as well as engage in some regular weight-bearing exercise. Many physicians also advocate estrogen-replacement therapy for post-menopausal women, specifically as a protection against osteoporosis, although estrogen supplementation is not without its drawbacks. There are also other nonhormonal medications that have become available over the last decade.

How does osteoporosis happen?

Among myriad potential causes, osteoporosis is believed most frequently to arise not from advancing disease, but from deficiency. In the 1980s, an expert panel assembled by the National Institutes of Health to investigate osteoporosis causes concluded specifically, "Among the many possible etiologies of primary osteoporosis, current data point to two probable causes: deficiency of estrogen and deficiency of calcium."

Why estrogen? Rapid bone loss often accompanies menopause, and removal of the ovaries results in premature osteoporosis. In both cases, estrogen replacement prevents bone loss.

Regarding the role that calcium deficiency plays in osteoporosis, the panel noted that in animal experiments, calcium deficiency caused osteoporosis; that low calcium intake is common among the elderly (and across all ages) in the United States; and that supplementation of calcium reduces bone loss.

Bones are made in part of calcium, but calcium serves a host of other functions in the body. When systemic needs are not met from outside calcium sources, the versatile human body fetches calcium from the bones, borrowing it for day-to-day existence. The once-dense structure of femurs and tibias morphs over time into a latticework of delicate bone lace, more and more resembling a coral formation than the strong support structure it once was.

The following figure illustrates the difference be-tween healthy bone and a bone affected by osteoporosis.

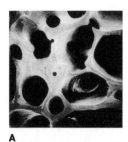

A

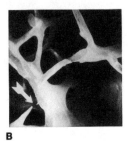

B

After menopause bones begin to break down, the need for calcium support becomes critical. But years of insufficient calcium intake before menopause may set up a situation in which the body is unable to play catch-up at a later date. Consequently, taking care of your bones from an early age is vitally important.

Boning up on bone

Bone is a natural matrix, rich in collagen, into which minerals are deposited—particularly calcium and phosphate. The types of bone are:

- Compact cortical bone, which makes up the outside walls of the skeleton
- Trabecular or medullary bone, which forms plates that stretch across the interior of the

skeleton (something like support beams in a building)

Different places in the body have different proportions of these two kinds of bones. Along the spine, for example, the second type dominates, but the thigh bone is mostly made of the first type. The distinction between types is important because each type has its own metabolic characteristics and susceptibility to fracture.

Although the skeleton is popularly used as a symbol of death, bone actually is living tissue that's constantly changing. Osteoclasts reabsorb bone in minuscule cavities; then osteoblasts restructure bone surfaces to smooth out the cavities. How this happens is a matter not only of mechanics, but also of electrical forces, hormones, and factors ranging from diet and digestion to kidney function.

Bones are at their best—that is to say, peak bone mass is achieved—for most people at around age 35. (That age applies to cortical bone; trabecular-bone mass peaks earlier.) The peak state depends on factors including gender, race, nutrition, level of physical activity, and overall health.

Bone mass increases most significantly from puberty until age 20. This is a critical time in a woman's life with respect to "boning up" on bone. The rate of increase in bone mass continues to increase at a slower rate until the mid thirties, when it peaks. From the moment that bone reaches its pinnacle, it begins slacking off in the remodeling department and gradually loses its mass throughout the rest of life. Not only the calcium and phosphorous deposits go, but also the organic matrix itself. The rate of bone loss speeds in women for three to seven years after menopause if measures are not taken to prevent its loss.

Watch Out!
Hip, wrist, and spine fractures are among the most common fractures attributable to osteoporosis.

Bone strength in the menopausal years ultimately depends on two factors: the peak bone mass from which a woman is starting at menopause and the rate of subsequent loss with each passing year after menopause. Factors that decrease the early accumulation of bone mass during the first four decades of life (such as low calcium intake, low body weight, anorexia nervosa, lack of estrogen, disease states that prevent proper absorption of nutrients from the intestines, and inactivity) will result in a less than optimal starting point at menopause. This sets the stage for osteopenia and subsequent osteoporosis.

Here are some more bone facts:

- Osteopenia is a pre-osteoporosis condition that indicates significant bone weakness and a predisposition for osteoporosis. It correlates with a bone mass that is 20 percent less than that in a 35-year-old woman (the peak bone-mass age).

- Osteoporosis is a condition in which the bone is so fragile that fractures occur even with minimal trauma.

- After peak bone mass is achieved at age 35, bone is then lost at 0.3 to 0.5 percent per year until menopause. After menopause there is an increased rate of bone loss at 2.3 percent for the next 6 years. Bone loss rate then decreases more slowly.

- Estrogen receptors have been identified in bone.

Who's at risk of developing osteoporosis?

Increased risk of developing osteoporosis depends on the following factors:

- Family history of osteoporosis.
- Age. The older you are, the greater your risk.
- Frame size and weight. The thinner and smaller you are, the greater your risk.
- Ethnicity. Caucasian and Asian women are in a higher risk category than are women of other races.
- Age at which menopause begins. Early onset of natural or surgically induced menopause increases your risk.
- Smoking. It increases your risk.
- Level of activity. The less exercise you get, the greater your risk.
- Disease. Stress to the system can increase risk, and thyroid and adrenal overactivity may result in calcium leaching.
- Some medications.
- Excessive alcohol use.
- History of anorexia nervosa.

Unofficially...
Women experience more fractures than men, and whites more than blacks.

Chemotherapy can provoke early menopause and increase osteoporosis risk. Other medications that may heighten risk (usually through interference with calcium absorption) are cortisone and other corticosteroids, thyroid hormone, anticonvulsants, diuretics, and antacids that contain aluminum. Caffeine and some foods can interfere with calcium absorption, too.

Can I tell whether I have osteoporosis?

Osteoporosis doesn't have outward signs during its early development, but with the help of a health professional, you can find out how your bones are doing. If you fit several risk factors or otherwise suspect osteoporosis, ask your physician about scheduling a bone-densitometry test, which is similar to an X-ray. In addition, a urine test called Osteomark can help gauge the rate of bone loss in cases in which dangerously rapid depletion is suspected.

If you're a postmenopausal woman at least 50 years old, Quiz 6.1 can help you determine whether you should ask for a bone-density (DEXA) scan.

As we've gained knowledge about the significance of bone strength with respect to menopause and aging, techniques for screening have improved. Screening can be useful in the following situations:

- To obtain a baseline bone density in order to assess an individual woman's risk of osteoporosis.

- As a way to follow bone strength once a treatment has been started, or if no treatment is used it can determine whether or not increased bone loss has occurred over time.

- It may be helpful in determining osteoporosis risk in women who want to change or stop treatment.

Tests that are useful for screening purposes should be accessible, accurate, and sensitive enough to detect small changes that occur over time in a slow process such as osteoporosis. Standard X-rays for example are *not* good screening tests since they lack the sensitivity needed. By the time evidence of osteoporosis is apparent on X-ray, 20 to 50 percent of bone mass has been lost. The following tests are currently available.

- Dual Energy X-ray Absorptiometry (DEXA): This is the most commonly used test to screen

QUIZ 6.1: SHOULD YOU ASK FOR A BONE-DENSITY SCAN?

1. Are you Caucasian, Hispanic, Asian, Native American/American Indian *or other than African American/Black*?

   (If yes, score 5 points)   _____

2. Do you take or have you ever taken hormone replacement therapy?

   (If no, score 1 point)   _____

3. Have you ever been treated for or told you have rheumatoid arthritis?

   (If yes, score 4 points)   _____

4. Since the age of 45, have you fractured a wrist, hip, or rib?

   (If yes, score 4 points for each of the three sites that you fractured)   _____

5. Take the first number of your age and multiply by 3 (67 years old = 6 × 3).   _____

6. Subtotal   _____

7. Divide your weight by 10, rounded off to the nearest whole number.   _____

8. Subtract item 7 from item 6.   _____

Score: If you score 6 or higher, you should discuss osteoporosis with your physician, as well as the possibility of scheduling a bone-density scan. (And if you scored under six, it's *still* a good idea to talk to your doctor about osteoporosis and the risk factors associated with it. Remember that while this quiz can be helpful, it's not a substitute for your physician's clinical judgment and consideration of any risk factors you may have.)

Source: Merck & Co., Inc. (SCORE - (Simple Calculated Osteoporosis Risk Estimation) test)

← Note!
In a test of 1,200 women, a score of 6 or higher was more than 80 percent accurate in predicting osteoporosis.

Watch Out!
Any woman over 50 who experiences a bone fracture from minimal trauma, such as a fall, should be suspected of having osteoporosis. A bone evaluation should be performed and it should include a DEXA scan.

for osteoporosis. It uses a small amount of radiation ($\frac{1}{20}$ of the dose of a standard chest X-ray) directed specifically at key areas of interest with respect to osteoporosis, that is areas with high levels of trabecular bone—the spine, the hip, and the wrist. It uses a computer to generate calculations of bone density and it is very accurate, measuring to within 5 percent of true bone density. The results are then calculated and reported as follows:

■ T score: A comparison with results expected for women at peak bone density (age 35).

■ Z score: A comparison with results expected for women of the same age as the person being tested.

A result that is 2 standard deviations lower than expected on the T score is consistent with osteopenia and values of more than 2.5 standard deviations loss is consistent with osteoporosis.

■ Quantitative Computed Tomography (QCT): This test uses X-ray techniques used in CAT scans. It measures the vertebral bodies of the spine. It uses a much greater amount of radiation and is a more expensive test. It is very accurate.

■ Single Photon Absorptiometry (SPA): This test is rarely used. It measures cortical bone and is therefore not particularly helpful when screening for osteoporosis.

■ Dual Photon Absorptiometry (DPA): This test measures both cortical and trabecular bone. It is not as sensitive as DEXA which is an improved version of this technique.

- Quantitative Ultrasound Densitometers: This is a new FDA approved technique to measure bone densitometry using sonogram (sound-wave) technology. It has the advantage of being easy to use and offers no radiation exposure. Since it is a new technique it is not widely available.

If osteoporosis is advanced, some outward signs may be apparent. Shrinking from your normal adult height can be due in part to osteoporosis, as can stooping due to "dowager's hump" (a curving spine), otherwise-unexplained backaches, and easy bone breakage.

Some types of fractures, such as those that involve compression of the vertebrae, can occur during routine activities such as bending, lifting, or just getting out of a chair or bed. Immediate, severe, local back pain often signals what's happened. Pain, however, doesn't accompany all vertebral fractures, some of which are detected only by X-rays. Loss of body height itself can indicate multiple vertebral fractures, and abdominal disorders (such as bloating and constipation) can also result.

Hip fractures, which are so common and frightening among the elderly, are particularly dangerous for their complications, not the least of which is depression resulting from the loss of mobility. Sadly, most hip-fracture patients never recover their normal activities again, and as mentioned earlier in this chapter, quite a few don't survive the year after their fracture occurs.

Osteoporosis isn't the only ailment that causes bone loss and thereby leads to risk of fracture. Following are some other conditions that can create bone loss:

- Certain hormone imbalances, such as gluco-cortoid excess, and thyroid or parathyroid imbalances

- Certain cancers, such as that of the bone marrow

- Osteomalacia (a disorder also known as adult-onset rickets, characterized by inadequate mineralization of bone)

Whenever you suspect excessive bone loss, it's important to investigate the possibility of metabolic bone diseases like those in the preceding list.

How do I prevent osteoporosis?

Remember that not everyone is destined to develop osteoporosis. One of the best ways to make sure that you're in the bone-healthy category is to take yourself *out* of high-risk categories (as much as possible) by doing the following things:

- If you smoke, stop.

- If you drink alcohol heavily, cut back or stop.

- If you're sedentary, start getting some regular weight-bearing exercise.

- Don't crash-diet.

- Follow other healthy-living precautions that may help keep you from premature menopause and, thus, increased osteoporosis risk.

- Review your medications with your physician to ensure that you've been offered options that don't increase osteoporosis risk. If you must take medications that leave you at risk of osteoporosis, discuss with your doctor taking extra precautions against osteoporosis as a concurrent therapy.

Beyond avoiding risk factors, you would do well to consider some of the following proactive measures against osteoporosis:

- Adequate calcium and vitamin D (among other nutrients)

- Estrogen-replacement therapy

- Fluoride (supplemented in water supplies and toothpastes)

- Medications that decrease bone resorption, such as biphosphonates and calcitonin.

Like many aspects of menopause treatment, osteoporosis preventatives and treatments include points of debate. A National Institutes of Health Consensus Statement on osteoporosis approaches summarizes how touchy an issue it can be:

"The appropriate timing and proper use of agents, such as calcium, vitamin D, estrogens, and fluorides, as well as the role of exercise are issues that have generated major research efforts and considerable controversy."

Chapter 7 summarizes the role of estrogen supplementation in preventing osteoporosis, and the chapter on nutrition addresses the critical role of calcium in preventing osteoporosis. As you'll find out, it's not as simple as just taking calcium; there's a delicate balance among that mineral, vitamin D, magnesium, and other nutrients.

Heart disease

After menopause, 70 percent of women develop cardiovascular disease. Coronary heart disease, which is the root of heart attacks, is the leading cause of death for American women. Each year twice as many women die from heart attacks as from all types of cancer combined. The importance of heart

Bright Idea
Look after your levels! Adequate estrogen, calcium, and vitamin D appear to play a role in preventing colorectal cancer as well as in preventing osteoporosis. And don't forget the importance of magnesium, boron, silicon, and zinc.

disease as the number one killer of women is not always appreciated by the general population or by the medical community. Studies show that only 8 percent of women in the general population consider themselves to be at increased risk of heart disease. Thus, women are less likely to identify themselves as being at increased risk of heart attack, to identify warning symptoms, and ultimately to seek medical care in a timely matter. Women with heart disease are more likely to die from a heart attack than their male counterparts. Obviously, heart disease is a very serious issue for females, although we have traditionally enjoyed a lower risk for cardiovascular problems in comparison with men.

Recent studies show estrogen to be a very powerful agent with potent heart-protecting properties. In fact, women who go through an early menopause (prior to age 45) or who go through an abrupt menopause through surgery are at an increased risk of coronary heart disease. It's interesting to note that women who go through menopause early (thus experiencing reduced levels of estrogens and other female sex hormones) lose their advantage over men in risk of coronary artery disease. It has long been appreciated that prior to menopause women had fewer heart attacks than men. Once menopause occurs and estrogen levels decrease, the advantage that women have over men evaporates over the course of 10 years.

Hormone replacement therapy has been shown in many studies to decrease the incidence of coronary heart disease by 50 percent! This is very exciting news for women and for medicine in general. Estrogen exerts its protective effects in many ways. One early finding was its beneficial effect on cholesterol levels. Estrogen decreases the "bad" cholesterol, LDL, by approximately 15 percent while it increases the "good" cholesterol, HDL, by approximately the same amount. Estrogen also has non-lipid effects that are very beneficial to the heart and to circulation in general. It has been shown to lower vascular resistance, which means it opens up the blood vessels and allows more blood to flow. Experi-ments have been performed during angiograms (X-ray tests that show the flow of blood through heart blood vessels) before and after the addition of estrogen to the bloodstream. Estrogen dramatically increased the diameter of the blood vessels as well as the blood flow. Estrogen also lowers other harmful blood components such as fibrino-gen, plasminogen activator inhibitor-1, and possibly homocysteine. These agents appear to promote plaque formation in blood vessels.

Menopause and advancing age seem to turn the tables on our inborn protection from heart disease. Risk in this department is definitely not for men only. After menopause, women's risk of death from heart disease increases. In fact, the American Heart Association reports that at older ages, women who have heart attacks are twice as likely as men to die from them within a few weeks.

Many things set you up for potential heart problems in later life, some of them preventable and some not. You can take the following quiz, adapted from American Heart Association guidelines, to help assess your own risk of heart attack and stroke.

You can't change some risk factors, such as your age and family health history. About 80 percent of people who die of coronary heart disease are 65 or older. Men run a greater risk of heart attacks than women do, and they tend to experience them earlier in life.

Unofficially...
Multiple medical studies show that estrogen reduces LDL (bad) cholesterol while it increases HDL (good) cholesterol.

QUIZ 6.2: ARE YOU AT RISK FOR HEART ATTACK OR STROKE?

1. Are you a woman over the age of 55?

2. Have you gone through menopause or had your ovaries surgically removed?

3. Has a close blood relative suffered a heart attack at a young age (before 55 if father or brother; before 65 if mother or sister)?

4. Has a close blood relative had a stroke?

5. Do you smoke, work daily with smokers, or live with a smoker?

6. Is your total cholesterol level 240 mg/dL or higher?

7. Is your HDL ("good") cholesterol level less than 35 mg/dL?

8. Do you not know your total cholesterol or HDL levels?

9. Is your blood pressure 140/90 mm Hg or higher, or have you have been told that your blood pressure is too high?

10. Do you not know what your blood pressure is?

11. Do you get less than half an hour of physical activity at least three days per week?

12. Are you 20 pounds overweight or more?

13. Do you have diabetes or otherwise need medicine to control blood sugar?

14. Have you had a heart attack, or do you have coronary-artery disease?

15. Have you been told that you have carotid-artery disease, or have you had a stroke?

16. Do you have an abnormal heartbeat?

Answers: Every *yes* answer means that you could run increased risk of heart attack or stroke. Be sure to discuss these factors with your doctor, and take steps in your daily life to protect against heart disease. If you don't know your blood pressure or cholesterol level, have it checked!

Source: Source: American Heart Association (Adapted from AHA Health Risk Awareness assessment)

If your parents had heart disease, you may be predisposed to suffer it as well. If you're African American, keep in mind that statistically, you have a higher risk of severe hypertension than whites, and therefore a greater chance of developing heart disease.

No matter what your age or family background, you can definitely avoid some risk factors, such as smoking. Smokers have more than twice the risk of heart attack as nonsmokers, and cigarette smoking is the largest risk factor for sudden cardiac death—double to four times the risk of nonsmokers. You've heard that secondhand smoke—the kind that you breathe when people around you are smoking—is dangerous. According to the American Heart Association, chronic exposure may also increase the risk of heart disease.

Beware of combining preventable risks, too. Risk of heart disease goes up along with cholesterol levels, but when other factors are present (such as high blood pressure and cigarette smoke), the risk increase is even greater. Combine high blood pressure with obesity, smoking, high cholesterol, diabetes, or inactivity and the risk of heart attack or stroke goes up severalfold.

Risk factors for heart problems and stroke include those listed in Table 6.1.

Diabetes appears to play a significant role in women's development of heart disease. Oddly enough, women who have diabetes have double the risk of heart disease of men who have diabetes. High triglycerides and low levels of so-called good cholesterol also seem to have a more pronounced risk effect in females compared with males.

Unofficially...
Do periods provide protection? Iron, which is thought to play a role in the development of heart disease, is lost during monthly menstrual bleeding and thus may reduce women's risk of heart disease.

TABLE 6.1: HEART AND STROKE RISK FACTORS

What You Can't Change	What You Can Change
Increasing age (and menopause)	Smoking
Gender (men are more likely to have problems)	High total cholesterol levels and low HDL cholesterol
Inherited family and ethnic-group risk	High blood pressure
	High blood triglycerides
	Physical inactivity
	Overweight
	Diabetes
	Responses to stress
	Lack of fiber in the diet
	Vitamin C deficiency
	High uric-acid levels
	High homocysteine levels
	Blood viscosity
	Suboptimal nutrition
	Use of birth-control pills (if you smoke)

Hormone use is also linked to heart disease. Paradoxically, however, oral contraceptives potentially increase heart disease risk, whereas hormone-replacement therapy apparently provides protection from heart disease. Chapter 7 sorts out that dilemma by discussing the pros and cons of hormone replacement.

Many residual concerns regarding the effect of HRT involve earlier observations that *high dose* oral contraceptive pills increased the risk of heart attack in women over age 35. Another study, the Coronary Drug Project, looked at the effect of *high dose* estrogen in men and found that it increased the risk of heart attack and blood clots. When we use HRT, we are using dosages many times lower than that found in early birth control pills.

Cancer

Cancer is a frightening specter, but despite its prevalence, it should not be women's No. 1 worry. Nearly twice as many women in the United States die of heart disease and stroke as die from all forms of cancer, including breast cancer.

Perhaps we fear cancer so much because it seems to be an invasion of our bodies, in which abnormal cells are growing out of control. The degeneration and imbalances that occur in heart disease and stroke may strike us as being a consequence of age. Many risk factors can be erased, however, and disease is hardly normal, no matter how widespread it is.

Does menopause play a role in cancer? In some ways, yes. We know that the occurrence of cancer increases as people age, that most cases affect adults who are middle-aged or older, and that some cancers are specifically related to age at menopause. Estrogen's role in the development of cancer also means that women whose hormone levels fluctuate greatly during perimenopause and menopause would do well to heed cancer-screening recommendations and take other preventative measures.

Estrogen is known to be linked to breast cancer and endometrial cancer, so these types of cancer are an issue in hormone-replacement therapy. Chapter 7 tackles this topic in detail.

Breast cancer

Breast cancer is the second-most-deadly cancer among women in the United States, claiming the lives of more than 45,000 females every year. About

Bright Idea
Get serious about good nutrition—it could save your life. Evidence suggests up to one-third of the 564,800 cancer deaths that are expected to occur in the United States this year are related to nutrition, according to the American Cancer Society.

183,000 new cases are diagnosed each year. Breast-cancer risk increases with age and has become a major point of debate in the advisability of hormone-replacement therapy, given estrogen's role in breast-tissue proliferation.

Breast cancer is also a menopausal issue for other reasons. The risk of breast cancer increases with age, and higher risk is also associated with women who have their first menstrual periods earlier than normal and go through menopause later than normal. It's suggested that the longer high levels of estrogens remain in the system, the greater a woman's predisposition to breast cancer is.

Risk factors for breast cancer, according to the American Cancer Society, include the following:

- Advancing age
- Personal or family history of breast cancer
- Biopsy-confirmed atypical hyperplasia
- Early menarche
- Late menopause
- Recent use of oral contraceptives or post-menopausal estrogens
- Never having had children or having the first live birth at a late age
- Higher education and socioeconomic status

Scientists continue to look into other factors that may contribute to breast-cancer risk, such as intake of fat and alcohol, exposure to pesticides and other chemicals, weight gain, induced abortion, and lack of exercise, as well as genetic influences. Recent studies have identified genes called BRCA1 and BRCA2 that are associated with 5-10 percent of breast cancers. Women that carry these genes have approximately 80 percent lifetime chance of developing breast cancer. These women are also at increased risk of getting ovarian cancer. Smoking has also been shown to increase the risk of all cancers in certain susceptible individuals who have a genetic defect in their ability to detoxify substances. Future research is ongoing.

Table 6.2 shows women's risk of breast cancer by age.

TABLE 6.2: WOMEN'S CHANCE OF DEVELOPING BREAST CANCER

Age Range	Chance of Developing Breast Cancer
By age 30	1 in 2,525
By age 40	1 in 217
By age 50	1 in 50
By age 60	1 in 24
By age 70	1 in 14
By age 80	1 in 10

Source: National Cancer Institute Surveillance Program.

The first sign of breast cancer typically is an abnormality that is visible on a mammogram. As the cancer grows, it often manifests itself as a breast lump, thickening, swelling, distortion, tenderness, skin irritation, or dimpling. Changes in nipple sensation and shape can also occur, although benign conditions are usually responsible for breast pain.

The National Institutes of Health recommends that all women 40 and older have regular mammograms (special X-ray pictures of the breast) and clinical breast exams, and the National Cancer Institute recommends frequent breast self-exams—many women check their breasts monthly. Mammograms are designed to find cancer in the earliest stages—even before lumps or any other symptoms develop. With early detection, 90 percent

Unofficially... Mammography may detect breast cancer up to two years before a lump can even be felt. In mammography, the breast is placed between plastic plates; a little pressure is applied to flatten it slightly, so as to get a clear picture. Mammography takes just a few minutes and should involve minimal discomfort.

of women who have breast cancer can be successfully treated.

Table 6.3 provides guidelines on how often you should consider breast-cancer screening.

Note! ➜
These guidelines apply to women who have no signs of breast cancer, such as a lump, breast distortion, or bloody nipple discharge. If you have any of these signs contact your doctor immediately.

TABLE 6.3: RECOMMENDED BREAST-CANCER SCREENING

Screening Method	Recommended Frequency of Screening
Mammograms	Age 40–49: every 1–2 years
	Over age 50: every year
Clinical breast exam	Annually, performed by your doctor
Self-exam	Monthly

Many women fail to get mammograms because they fear the small amount of radiation used in the mammogram will induce a cancer. The statistical risk of this happening is much less than 1 percent, which is a negligible risk when one considers the lifesaving benefits of early detection. Remember that over 90 percent of women who detect cancers less than ½ inch in size, smaller than the size often detected with mammograms, survive.

Uterine cancer

About 36,100 cases of uterine cancer (usually, cancer of the endometrium) are diagnosed every year, and 6,300 deaths are expected as a result of this cancer, according to the American Cancer Society.

Abnormal uterine bleeding or spotting is a chief sign of uterine cancer. Pain and systemwide problems don't usually develop until the disease has progressed. The major risk factor is estrogen.

Increased risk of uterine cancer is likely for women who:

▪ Are on estrogen-replacement therapy without a progestin supplement

- Are taking tamoxifen
- Began having periods at an early age
- Entered menopause late
- Have never had children
- Have a history of failure to ovulate
- Have diabetes, gallbladder disease, or hypertension, or are obese

Unofficially...
Adding a progestin to estrogen-replacement therapy seems to have protective effects, similar to those of pregnancy and the use of oral contraceptives.

When women reach 40 years of age, they are advised to have an annual pelvic exam. Pap smears, which are greatly effective in detecting cervical cancer early, are rarely effective in detecting endometrial cancer. At menopause an endometrial biopsy is recommended for those women who have abnormal unexplained bleeding or who have high risk factors for developing this type of cancer. This office procedure is simple to perform and effective to screen those at risk. Early detection in this way makes this one of the most successfully treated malignancies.

Colo-rectal cancer

Colo-rectal cancer is the second-most-diagnosed cancer, the No. 2 cause of cancer death in Western nations, and the No. 3 cause of cancer deaths in American women. About 150,000 new cases are diagnosed in the United States annually, and an estimated 7 percent of Americans will develop colo-rectal cancer.

Risk factors include family history of colo-rectal cancer; smoking; poor, low-fiber diet; lack of physical activity; and excessive weight. If colon cancer is detected in its early stages, patients have a long-term survival rate of 91 percent.

Because of the increased risk brought on by age, a colo-rectal cancer test is recommended twice a decade after age 50, Home tests are also available, but they shouldn't replace a trip to the doctor.

Increased calcium and Vitamin D intake may decrease the risk of colo-rectal cancer (see Chapter 10).

Screening for cancer

The American Cancer Society recommends that women who don't show specific cancer symptoms still take part in early-detection testing. Table 6.4 summarizes current guidelines on who should be tested for what and how often.

Moneysaver
Free colo-rectal-cancer screenings are often available at health fairs held by hospitals. Ask your local hospital's public-affairs department or your local wellness center for information.

Note! ➜
These screening recommendations are for people who show no symptoms. If you have symptoms of any of these cancers or are in a particularly high risk group, your physician may advise more-frequent screening or additional tests.

TABLE 6.4: CANCER SCREENING

Screening Method	Frequency
Cancer-related checkups	A cancer-related checkup is recommended every 3 years for people ages 20 to 40 and every year for people age 40 and older. This exam should include health counseling. Depending on a person's age, the exam may include examinations for cancers of the thyroid, oral cavity, skin, lymph nodes, and ovaries, as well as for some nonmalignant diseases.
Breast exams	Women age 40 and older should have an annual mammogram and an annual clinical breast exam (CBE) performed by a health-care professional; they also should perform monthly self-examination. The CBE should be conducted close to the time of the scheduled mammogram. Women ages 20 to 39 should have a CBE every three years and should perform monthly breast self examination.
Colon and rectum exams	Women age 50 and older should follow one of the following exam schedules*:
	—Fecal occult blood test every year and flexible sigmoidoscopy every five years

	—Colonoscopy every 10 years; Double-contrast barium enema every 5 to 10 years.
	—Digital rectal exam at the same time as the sigmoidoscopy, colonoscopy, or double-contrast barium enema.
Uterus and cervix exams	All women who are (or have been) sexually active or who are age 18 and older should have an annual Pap test and pelvic examination. After three or more consecutive satisfactory examinations with normal findings, the Pap test may be performed less frequently. Discuss the matter with your physician.
Endometrium exams	Women who are at high risk for cancer of the uterus should have a sample of endometrial tissue examined when menopause begins.

* People who are at moderate or high risk for colo-rectal cancer should talk with a doctor about setting up a different testing schedule.

Source: American Cancer Society

Screening can detect cancers of the breast, colon, rectum, cervix, tongue, mouth, and skin at early stages in women. Along with screening for cancer of the prostate and testes in men, these screenable cancers account for about half of all new cancer cases, according to the American Cancer Society. Overall, the relative five-year survival rate for these types of cancer is around 80 percent. Health experts suggest that if all Americans had regular screenings, that survival rate could move up to more than 90 percent.

Alzheimer's disease

Another ailment that has links to menopause is Alzheimer's disease. The symptoms of this disease

Timesaver
The Alzheimer's Association can provide a wealth of information on this disease, including a booklet on women and Alzheimer's disease. You can get a copy of the booklet by completing an online request form (www.alz.org) or by calling (800) 272-3900.

(which is not fully understood) include memory loss and general senility. As many as one of every three families must cope with Alzheimer's disease, which is a slowly debilitating condition that affects about 4 million people in the United States—and three times as many women as men. The majority of Alzheimer's patients are 65 or older. Alzheimer's disease has no known cure, but considerable efforts to develop treatments are under way.

Why is Alzheimer's associated with menopause? Several medical studies have found that estrogen enhances memory, and in some cases, memory loss can be associated with a lack of estrogen. Hormone-replacement therapy has had dramatic protective effects in some studies in this arena, as discussed in Chapter 7.

Table 6.5 shows your overall risk of developing Alzheimer's disease.

TABLE 6.5: ALZHEIMER'S RISK BY AGE

Age	Chance of Developing Alzheimer's Disease
65	10%
75	20%
85	40–50%

People whose family members have had Alzheimer's may be predisposed to develop the disease themselves. Clearly, low estrogen levels can also play a role. There may be an environmental connection as well; unusually high levels of aluminum have been found in the brains of Alzheimer's patients. Scientists are still studying what other things may contribute to risk factors. Among the topics of research are strokes, head injuries, and infections.

Physicians can diagnose Alzheimer's disease with considerable accuracy by reviewing patients' family and personal histories, as well as by conducting brain scans, laboratory tests, and various question-and-answer tests. After a diagnosis of Alzheimer's is made, a physician can order a blood test that identifies a gene implying increased risk. But this test is not conclusive. Some people who have the gene don't get Alzheimer's, and some people who have Alzheimer's don't have the gene. Alzheimer's disease is an area of active research, and you can expect additional diagnosis and treatment methods in years to come.

Alzheimer's disease may take about 7 years to develop fully but has been known to take up to 20 years to reach its final stages. Symptoms include a progression of the following:

- Memory loss

- Confusion

- Difficulty completing routine tasks

- Disorientation

- Personality changes

- Poor judgment

- Difficulty feeding or bathing oneself

- Anxiety

- Altered sleeping patterns

- Speech and recognition difficulties (inability to recognize even family members and close friends)

- Increasing dependency on others for routine care

Bright Idea
The herb ginkgo biloba has been extensively studied for its positive implications for Alzheimer's. Vitamin E may also slow the progression of the disease.

Stroke, head injury, alcohol consumption, depression, infection, and family history have been studied as possible links to Alzheimer's, but the evidence is inconclusive. New drugs have been approved for the treatment of Alzheimer's. And some over-the-counter medications, as well as herbs and vitamins, may prevent or slow the disease.

Most of the information we have on risks and benefits of HRT with respect to heart disease and cancer is the product of retrospective studies. These are studies that take data via observations of events that have already occurred. While very informative, these studies are not as compelling as prospective studies. Prospective studies evaluate information and outcomes as they occur. These studies are difficult and expensive to run because they need to take place over a prolonged period of time and need to include a large cohort of people in order to give meaningful results. To date only one large study, the Postmenopausal Estrogen/Progestin Intervention Trial (PEPI), has been completed. It showed a decrease in mortality due to heart disease by 50 percent in users of HRT. It did not give definitive results with respect to breast cancer risk. Some ongoing prospective studies designed to investigate the effect of HRT on development of heart disease and of breast cancer currently underway are:

- Women's Health Initiative
- Heart and Estrogen-Progestin Replacement Study (HERS)
- Women's International Study of long Duration Oestrogen after Menopause (WISDOM)
- Million Women Study

The results of these studies will be crucial in getting solid data on the risks and benefits of HRT on critical issues that affect women's health. They will be anxiously awaited by everyone involved in women's health issues.

Just the facts

- Osteoporosis is largely attributed to a deficiency of estrogen or calcium.

- Seven of every 10 postmenopausal women stand to develop cardiovascular disease.

- Mammography can detect breast cancer up to two years before symptoms develop.

- Women make up 72 percent of the U.S. population age 85 and older, and nearly half this group has Alzheimer's disease.

- Alzheimer's disease is associated, in some cases, with estrogen deficiency.

Hormone Treatments

GET THE SCOOP ON...
What hormones are replaced in HRT ▪
The debate over HRT and cancer ▪
What conditions HRT can help prevent ▪
Why women refuse or discontinue HRT

PART III

Hormone-Replacement Therapy (HRT)

Chapter 7

S ay "menopause treatment," and what comes to mind? Probably estrogen replacement. Hormonal decline brings on menopause. Supplementation—primarily of the sex hormone estrogen but also of progesterone (usually with synthetic progestins)—and sometimes testosterone is viewed by many as being a way to bring hormones back to previous levels, stay youthful, and fend off disease that *might* otherwise occur.

The major female sex hormones, estrogen and progesterone, are powerful substances. Before birth, they allowed you to develop female features instead of male ones. At puberty, they were responsible for the growth of your breasts and the onset of your menstrual periods. And if you're a mother, you couldn't have become one without them.

Replacing these declining hormones may seem to be a natural way to ensure continuing health, but the powerful effects that make them so useful also make them touchy to work with in many cases—and

Unofficially...
Can estrogen keep you looking young? In studies of hormone-therapy patients, estrogens appeared to increase the collagen content of the skin, and in a study of more than 3,000 women, wrinkling and dryness appeared to be decreased in patients who had used estrogen.

sometimes even possibly dangerous. The benefits of replacement are great, but replacement is not without potential risks. This chapter describes both the benefits and the risks of hormone replacement-therapy (HRT).

A little hormone history

Extracts of animal sex glands have been used in the treatment of gynecological disorders for centuries. But it wasn't until the late 1920s that scientists isolated the hormone estrogen, and in the next decade, they isolated progesterone. At that time, it was known that hormones could prevent animals from ovulating, but much remained to be discovered. Researchers focused on the new development, and by 1940, many studies had been published on the relationship of hormones to diseases such as cancer.

The development of hormone-replacement therapy went hand in hand with the rise of the birth-control pill. The treatments are similar, after all; they are simply used for different purposes. Margaret Sanger, a nurse who became an early women's-rights activist and the founder of Planned Parenthood, crusaded for an effective, inexpensive method of birth control. Her search led her, at near the age of 90, to a scientist named Gregory Pincus. Sanger raised about $150,000 to get Pincus started on research that, in combination with the work of other scientists, led to the development of the birth-control pill.

Because several scientific studies had associated estrogen with cancer, Pincus and another researcher, Dr. Min Cheuh Chang, focused on progesterone, the other major female sex hormone. They collaborated with a Harvard gynecologist named Dr. John Rock, who was using hormones in experimental infertility treatment. In 1948 Pincus was awarded a small grant from Planned Parenthood Federation of America to test steroids for their contraceptive value. Additional funding for the project was sought and by the mid-1950s the group began contraceptive-pill tests on humans. In 1960 the Food and Drug Administration approved the sale of steroid pills for contraception.

During the 1950s, the benefits of estrogen for menopausal women started to become known. The hormone was widely promoted by the medical community, and large numbers of women started taking it , for reasons that ranged from alleviating their hot flashes to preserving their beauty past menopause. Yet few women had heard about the potential drawbacks of estrogen-replacement therapy—particularly the possible association of estrogen with the development of cancer.

A new crop of reports questioning the wisdom of estrogen-replacement therapy arose in the mid-1970s. Several study findings paired estrogen use after menopause with an endometrial-cancer rate up to eight times the norm. (*Endometrial cancer* is cancer of the uterine lining.) The backlash against hormones had begun, and estrogen use dropped as physicians hesitated at the prescription pad.

At that point, the *progesterone* side of things began to gain the attention of researchers. Studies found that adding a synthetic form of progesterone (a progestin) to estrogen-replacement regimens *protected* women against endometrial cancer. The idea of replacing hormones regained popularity, and by 1994, approximately 40 percent of menopausal women in the United States were undergoing hormone replacement therapy.

> **"** In the last 30 years, we have made enormous advances in understanding how estrogen works in multiple physiologic systems and how much it affects the health of aging women. We have also made major improvements in how we prescribe estrogen.—Dr. Bruce Ettinger, Division of Research, Kaiser Permanente Medical Care Program; "Overview of Estrogen Replacement Therapy: A Historical Perspective"; Proceedings of the Society for Experimental Biology and Medicine, 217(1):2-5 1998 Jan **"**

Unofficially...
Recent studies reported by Jonathan Baron, Ph.D.; Gerald B. Holzman, M.D.; and Jay Schulkin, Ph.D., for the American College of Obstetricians and Gynecologists suggest that hormone-replacement therapy may reduce tooth loss, colon cancer, and loss of brain function.

HRT today

Hormone-replacement therapy has found a huge number of proponents in medicine. Some physicians and scientists call it perhaps the most important development in preventive medicine in the Western world for half a century. A large number of studies of hormone replacement suggest that for most women, the benefits outweigh the risks. These benefits include cardiovascular and bone protection, reduction or elimination of hot flashes and insomnia, and improvement of energy and mood.

But drawbacks—largely having to do with cancer risk—are still a matter of great controversy, not to mention research, as the need for good long-term data is voiced again and again. Also, cautionary critics remind us that *slightly healthier women may take menopausal* hormones to begin with, which could influence the results of any studies that do not specifically account for it. In a study of more than 500 women followed through menopause, University of Pittsburgh researchers found those who wound up using estrogen tended to be thinner and were more likely to have had oral contraceptive use in their history than non-estrogen users.

Despite the benefits of HRT in alleviating certain symptoms of difficult menopause and protecting against serious health disorders, a survey conducted by Dr. Philip Sarrel, professor of obstetrics/gynecology and psychiatry at the Yale University School of Medicine, estimates that only 8 percent to 12 percent of postmenopausal women undergo replacement therapy for two years or longer. Most women, therefore, do not undergo the therapy long enough to gain protection against osteoporosis and heart disease.

For substantial osteoporosis prevention, Framingham study data suggests its necessary to take estrogen for at least seven years. The greatest benefits in preventing heart disease are also seen with *long-term* use. A 1991 study found estrogen replacement cut the risk of death from cardiovascular disease by almost half—when women were on it for 15 years.

But the great majority of women are not committing to anything resembling a long-term regimen. In fact, a 1996 study done for the Lister Hospital in Great Britain reported that up to 75 percent of women who started HRT dropped out within the first six months (and many women don't even fill the HRT prescriptions their doctors write for them).

Sarrel's survey, which included 252 perimenopausal and postmenopausal women participating in the Prime Plus menopause support group, suggested these reasons for taking HRT:

1. To control symptoms (77 percent)

2. To prevent osteoporosis (73 percent)

3. To prevent heart disease (55 percent)

4. To maintain sexual function (41 percent)

5. To prevent stroke (37 percent)

6. To prevent Alzheimer's disease (32 percent)

The survey also found that when women decide against HRT, they tend to do so for the following reasons:

1. Bleeding (34 percent)

2. Fear of cancer (17 percent—a figure that increases to 22 percent among perimenopausal women)

Timesaver
There are ways to protect bone health beyond estrogen supplementation. Some evidence exists that androgens (such as testosterone) may help preserve bone mass, too. New treatment options include alendronate (Fosamax) and calcitonin (Miacalcin). Adequate calcium and vitamin D are important, of course.

3. Weight gain (14 percent)

4. Failure to control symptoms (12 percent)

Recent studies have made headway in refuting the commonly held suspicion that HRT causes weight gain. Larger weight gains have occurred in patients who were taking placebos than in those who actually received estrogen therapy or a combined estrogen–progestin regimen. One study of women in estrogen-receiving groups showed that over the course of more than three years of therapy, the women gained a little weight, on average, but women on placebos gained much more.

These findings support the idea that menopause (or at least aging) sometimes goes hand in hand with rising weight levels. When researchers looked at body-fat distribution, they found that therapy including a progestin was associated with a slight increase in the total fat percentage of the abdomen, but that this increase was less than a fifth of the increase that occurred in placebo groups.

Yet what happens to a group of women in a controlled trial does not account for individual biochemistry. Time and again, women who discuss their menopause and HRT experiences say that weight gain played a role. Are they incorrectly attributing to hormone regimens the weight gain that would have occurred without replacement therapy? In some cases, yes. But many types of estrogen and progestin (or progesterone) are available, and tinkering with type and dosage can make the difference between night and day for some women who are sensitive to HRT—not only in terms of weight and other side effects, but also in terms of the intended benefits of the program. This is one area in which working with an astute, caring physician

Bright Idea
Certain herbs may help relieve menopausal symptoms. In a 1991 German study, women with common menopause-related psychological symptoms were tracked for eight weeks. Those who received the Polynesian herb kava kava instead of a placebo reported reduced severity of symptoms, less depression, and a greater sense of general well-being.

can dramatically improve the quality of your therapeutic experience. Don't settle for less.

The decision to try HRT is not an easy one, but you have many options, some of which are likely to fit your needs better than others. And should you decide that HRT is not for you, you can still do a great deal to stay healthy and comfortable through menopause, through the use of good nutrition, herbs, exercise, and alternative health practices that allow many women to control their symptoms.

Variations: Just estrogen, or progesterone too?

Estrogen is still the most commonly prescribed hormone, although its combination with a progestin is thought to offer the most protection for women undergoing hormone-replacement therapy. This pairing most closely approximates what really happens in the cycling female body every month.

There are three typical forms of HRT:

- The use of estrogen by itself

- The use of estrogen throughout the month, with progestins added for part of the menstrual cycle

- The use of continuous estrogen and continuous progestins

Sometimes, androgens such as testosterone are added to HRT regimens. There are also new estrogen-like medicines that have recently become FDA approved that will be discussed later.

Hormone-replacement therapy may not be appropriate if there is a possibility of pregnancy, if you have breast or uterine cancer, liver disease, history of blood clots, undiagnosed abnormal vaginal bleeding, or uncontrolled hypertension. It should

Unofficially...
Women can take hormones in a variety of ways, including traditional pills, creams, and patches. The effects may differ, as you see in Chapter 8.

be used with caution in those women with genetic problems with lipid metabolism (familial hyper-lipoproteinemia). It can potentially be associated with fluid retention, which could worsen asthma, epilepsy, migraine, and heart or kidney dysfunction.

Lab tests can tell you whether your hormone levels are low enough that hormone therapy might be suggested. Ovarian failure is diagnosed in irregular menstruation or amenorrhea, when the blood serum FSH (Follicle Stimulating Hormone) levels are elevated (values above 50mIU/mL) and levels of estradiol (see the following section) are decreased (values under 50pg/mL). These values will vary from one lab to another—look for results out of normal range or ask your doctor for a more complete explanation of test values. The important thing is to see if the FSH is elevated *at the same time* that the estradiol level is low.

The decision to start HRT, however, should not take only lab tests into account—it is a complex matter that ultimately depends on the subjective opinions of both you and your doctor.

Estrogen-only therapy

As mentioned in earlier chapters, the term *estrogen* is a bit misleading, in that it refers to more than one hormone. The main estrogens made in the human body include those listed in Table 7.1.

There are many different forms of estrogen that can be used in estrogen replacement therapy. These medicines can be modified from natural sources or they can be formulated in the lab. The most frequently prescribed estrogen in the United States is sold under the brand name Premarin. Estrogenic compounds are isolated from the urine of pregnant horses and are modified by a chemical reaction

TABLE 7.1: THREE KINDS OF ESTROGEN IN A WOMAN'S BODY

estrone (also known as E1)	Made from estradiol, a "weak" estrogen; the main estrogen produced by the body after menopause
estradiol (also known as E2)	The primary estrogen; made in the ovaries
estriol (also known as E3)	A metabolite of estradiol; the estrogen that is prevalent during pregnancy; possibly protects against some cancers

← Note! Estradiol, the most prevalent estrogen made by the female body during fertile years, is also known as 17 beta-estradiol. It is the most potent form of estrogen that naturally occurs in the body.

called conjugation that allows the hormone to be absorbed by the body. These compounds are often referred to in the medical literature as *conjugated equine estrogens*. Most medical studies to date have used conjugated equine estrogens. Thus most of the information we have with respect to the side effects and benefits of HRT pertain specifically to this form of estrogen. With the interest rising in other forms of HRT more studies will be done on these compounds in the future.

There are many different estrogenic preparations available to women. They differ in their chemical composition as well as in the route of administration. The three main naturally occurring estrogens in the human body are estrone, estradiol, and estriol. The medicines used in HRT use preparations that are formulated in the lab from either plant sources, urine of pregnant animals, or totally synthetic precursors. "Natural" hormones are those that have the exact same chemical structure as those hormones found in the body. They are not necessarily made from plant sources although some of them are derived from these sources. It is unclear whether "natural" is better—further research is needed to determine the risks and benefits. Estradiol is the strongest estrogen, which may in fact be like a two edged sword. While it may offer the most benefit in terms of body response, it may also be the most likely to cause malignancy. Current research is focusing on the benefits of new estrogenic substances which bind selectively to estrogen receptors. These medicines show promise in giving estrogen benefits while actually reducing breast cancer rates.

There are several routes to administer hormones. They may be given orally in the form of a pill or capsule. They can be absorbed through mucus membranes via the vaginal or sublingual (under the tongue) routes; through skin (transdermally) via patches, pellets, or creams; and through muscle by way of intramuscular injection. Hormones given orally are first absorbed from the stomach and sent directly to the liver where further breakdown occurs. This "first pass effect" through the liver is felt to improve the lipid profile by decreasing the "bad" cholesterol, LDL. It also increases the risk (slightly) of gallstones since the gallbladder becomes more involved with the processing of hormones given orally. The vaginal route allows for more direct effects on the vagina, urinary bladder, and uterus. All routes allow hormones to enter the bloodstream in significant amounts.

Chapter 8 discusses the types of estrogens and their effects in detail.

Although Premarin is the most popular form of estrogen-replacement therapy in the United States, Europeans traditionally do things differently. In

Europe, estrogen-replacement therapy based on the natural human estrogen estriol is popular.

Combined estrogen and progesterone replacement

When the idea of hormone-replacement therapy took hold in the 1950s, estrogen was the only hormone that was typically supplemented. It wasn't until the 1970s, when the danger of unopposed estrogen—a significantly increased risk of endometrial cancer in those women with a uterus in place—became known. When it was shown in the 1980s in multiple medical studies that adding a progestin to the regimen would actually protect women from endometrial hyperplasia (a premalignant forerunner of endometrial cancer), combination hormone replacement therapy again became popular.

Today, *progestins*—synthetic forms of progesterone—are prescribed alongside estrogen in HRT because of their protective effect against cancer of the uterus. Progestins balance the proliferative effects of estrogen on the endometrium. When given in the proper dose, progestins prevent the development of endometrial hyperplasia and cancer that could result from estrogen-only therapy. There are several treatment regimens for progestin administration. They can be given in a cyclic manner, that is for 10 to 14 days per month, in which case monthly bleeding will usually occur. This bleeding is usually light and is predictable. Progestins can also be given continuously, every day along with estrogen, in which case they often cause no bleeding. Frequently this absence of bleeding (amenorrhea) may take several months to occur. When women are given a continuous regimen, they should be cautioned to expect some spotting or staining for the first 3 to 6 months. Bleeding at this point in therapy is not a cause for alarm, but it should be monitored by the physician. Some women never attain amenorrhea and may find cyclic therapy to be a better alternative. As in any instance of abnormal bleeding, endometrial biopsy in the doctor's office is sometimes needed to ensure that malignancy is not occuring.

It cannot be emphasized too strongly that the proper use of progestin with HRT will generally protect against endometrial cancer and that this form of cancer is not increased with combined estrogen and progestin therapy. While combination HRT has a minimal risk of inducing endometrial hyperplasia (well below 1 percent), it should be kept in mind that cancer can occur in any part of the body and persistent abnormal bleeding should be evaluated. For those women who have undergone hysterectomy the addition of a progestin is simply not needed. For these women many doctors believe estrogen-only therapy is preferable.

Progestins can be prescribed as a separate pills or in combination estrogen-progestin pills, such as those marketed as Prempro and Premphase. A new development is the arrival of the first combination estrogen and progestin transdermal patch, CombiPatch. In HRT, a progestin (or synthetic progesterone) is typically prescribed for women whose uteruses have not been surgically removed. But progestins may be medically unsafe or ill-advised in women who have had either liver disease or blood clots, as is estrogen therapy.

So, what is the problem with progestins? Historically, progestins haven't been well tolerated. They can cause bloating, weight gain, depression and moodiness, painful breasts, and unusual vaginal bleeding. They also may aggravate certain medical conditions, such as asthma, epilepsy, migraine headaches, and heart failure. Progestins when given in high doses will negate some of the beneficial effects estrogen has on cholesterol metabolism. They increase total cholesterol and LDL while reducing HDL.

The good news is that while progestins have a less favorable effect on cholesterol than estrogen, the net effects of estrogen on the cardiovascular system (namely improved cholesterol and lipid profile, increased diameter of blood vessels, decreased plaque formation, and antioxidant activity) are not offset by the addition of a progestin. The Postmenopausal Estrogen/Progestin Intervention (PEPI) study published in 1995 addressed this issue. They concluded that a combination of estrogen and progestin therapy can be used to prevent endometrial hyperplasia without interfering with the benefits of estrogen on the cardiovascular system.

Estrogen, progestin, and other replacement therapies

In addition to experiencing a decline in hormones associated with the reproduction system, many menopausal women may be low in other hormone levels, such as thyroid. And just as female-sex-hormone levels decrease at menopause, so do the levels of androgens—male hormones (androstenedione and testosterone) that the female body uses in minute quantities. Some physicians find that some of their menopausal patients benefit when testosterone is added to the HRT regimen.

Androgens are produced both in the ovaries and adrenal glands. Every day, women actually make more of these substances than they do estrogens, but most of the androgens that they produce are

Unofficially...
A recent Yale survey revealed interesting attitudes about hormone replacement. Although 98 percent of the women surveyed considered estrogen to be a natural hormone for the female body, and although 67 percent believed that progesterone is natural, fewer than half—46 percent—believed that testosterone (or androgen) is a natural hormone, and just 17 percent knew that androgens can prevent osteoporosis.

converted to estrogens. Androgens will often increase during the late perimenopause and early menopause years. They decrease to half these levels 10 years after the last menstrual period. Women who undergo removal of both their ovaries experience the most dramatic changes in androgen levels and often suffer the most severe symptoms. Since there are receptors for androgens throughout the body, these symptoms are not unexpected.

Along with helping prevent osteoporosis and possibly playing a role in stimulating new bone growth, androgens are strongly linked with libido. One study of postmenopausal women on estrogen who complained of sexual dysfunction reported an 80 percent improvement in libido when testosterone was added to hormone replacement.

When testosterone is prescribed as an adjunct in HRT, it's typically for women who have otherwise been unable to find relief from hot flashes or who find their sex drives lagging. Some physicians believe that lack of appropriate amounts of androgens can prompt more severe and frequent hot flashes; more and longer-lasting symptoms, due to urogenital atrophy; and greater frequency of psychological problems, such as depression. In certain cases, testosterone may also improve energy levels and mood.

There is, however, a downside to androgen-replacement therapy: the risk of unwanted side effects. Most notable among these side effects are acne and the growth of facial or body hair. Some women are more prone than others to develop these side effects. Also, hair growth, once stimulated may be permanent, requiring electrolysis for removal. These effects are usually not severe, however, since treatment can always be altered or discontinued if side effects occur. It should be kept in mind that if large amounts of testosterone are given over prolonged intervals, more masculinizing symptoms may be seen. These symptoms include deepened voice, hair loss on the scalp, increased muscle mass, or a masculine appearance. When testosterone replacement is given correctly, these effects should not be observed.

In HRT, androgens can be prescribed separately or in combination with estrogens. Two combination pills on the market today are Estratest and Estratest HS. When androgens are given orally in low dose, such as the dose present in EstraTest, there still is a positive effect on the heart due to estrogen. Your doctor can check androgen levels in your blood and help you decide whether adding androgens to your daily regimen is appropriate.

Risk or benefit?

On the whole, hormone-replacement therapy offers women the promise of relief from difficult menopausal experiences and protection from a batch of serious conditions to which they might otherwise be subject. But the potential risks posed by HRT are not to be taken lightly. In fact, the ongoing dilemma is how to ensure that the potential "cure" of replacement therapy isn't worse than the condition that it seeks to address. Also, HRT can cause unpleasant side effects: breast tenderness, fluid retention, occasionally aggravation of high blood pressure, monthly bleeding (depending on the type of regimen prescribed), nausea, and other discomforts.

As you must for any medical treatment, weigh the benefits of HRT against the negative factors. Much depends on getting the right regimen to work with your body.

Watch Out!
Therapy with androgens tends to cut production of the "good" cholesterol, HDL, thereby removing the benefit of estrogen supplementation's tendency to increase HDL levels.

Timesaver
Before you
decide on an
HRT regimen,
check Chapter 8,
which describes
how dosages and
types may
affect you.

In addition to helping relieve some of the typical symptoms of a difficult menopause, such as hot flashes and mood swings, estrogen protects bones against osteoporosis, and some studies show that it protects the heart as well. But the risks of estrogen-only therapy include an increased possibility of developing endometrial cancer and gallbladder disease. Although the addition of a progestin counters the additional endometrial-cancer risk, it may also cut the benefits that estrogen provides the heart. The slightly increased risk of breast cancer associated with long-term estrogen use is also a point of debate. Table 7.2 summarizes the pros and cons associated with estrogen in replacement therapy.

TABLE 7.2: PROS AND CONS OF ESTROGEN REPLACEMENT

Pros	Cons
Osteoporosis prevention: Helps maintain and replenish bone density.	Increased risk of endometrial cancer: occurs with prolonged estrogen therapy without a progestin in women with an intact uterus
Cardiovascular disease prevention: Reduces LDL cholesterol (the "bad" type) and increases HDL cholesterol (the "good" type).	Increased risk of gallbladder disease and gallstones Possibility of an increased risk of breast cancer.
Lowers blood pressure	
Reduces insulin levels	

Early estrogen alarm

Early experiences with estrogen supplementation were disastrous, to say the least. In England back in 1938, Sir Charles Dodds synthesized an estrogen that was both effective when taken orally and inexpensive to produce. That estrogen was diethylstilbestrol (DES).

Noticing that hormone levels were low in women who had miscarriages, doctors prescribed DES to help preserve pregnancies in women who were at high risk of miscarrying. Five to 10 million American women are believed to have received DES during pregnancy or to have been exposed to the drug before their own birth. But cancers were found to result in an unusually large number of children born to mothers who took the hormone during pregnancy. Some women, so-called DES daughters, who were exposed to DES before birth in the 1940s and '50s, developed cancer of the vagina and cervix in the 1960s and '70s. Exposure to DES was also associated with increased breast-cancer risk in DES mothers.

The lesson of DES is being taken seriously, and legions of studies involving estrogens are attempting to sort out which of them might promote cancer. No one can yet say unequivocally that all estrogens on the market are safe under all conditions. The decision to use estrogen in replacement therapy is one that you should make only after your own review of current knowledge, and only with your doctor's advice.

Hormones and cancer

Estrogen stimulates cell growth, as when the lining of the uterus is being built up during the first half of the menstrual cycle. The connection between estrogen-promoted cell proliferation and cancer is simple to see. Studies show that estrogen plays a role in stimulating unusually rapid growth of breast tissue. In the 1950s, scientists demonstrated that giving estrogens to lab rats produced breast tumors.

But studies of breast cancer development among HRT users have yielded conflicting results. Some of the risk appears time-dependent. Many researchers believe there's little or no increase in a woman's risk of breast cancer when she has used HRT for 10 years or less, but that she faces a moderately increased risk when HRT use exceeds 10 years.

The cancer potential posed by estrogen—even the estrogen that our own bodies manufacture—is a chief reason why progestins or progesterone are added to hormone replacement regimens. The addition of these substances balances the action of estrogen in the uterus. What they do in other areas of the body is less certain. A 1996 Swedish review suggests future research will be needed to define the long-term safety of various progestin regimens. While progestins are actually used in the *treatment* of some breast cancers, that's not the whole story. They've also been recently *implicated* in stimulating the development of some kinds of breast cancer cells. We'll say it again—there's much research yet to be done.

Earlier in this chapter we mentioned that despite the popularity of HRT women don't typically stay on it very long—not really long enough to get heart-protective or bone-protective effects of much magnitude. The flip side to the coin is the possibility of increased cancer risk from long-term use. An American Cancer Society study of 240,000 women found those taking estrogen 6 years or more experienced a 40 percent increased risk of fatal ovarian cancer. When women took estrogen 11 years or longer, the increase rose to 70 percent.

Some physicians suspect that fluctuating estrogen levels may also contribute to cancer risk during perimenopause, when the body's progesterone output diminishes due to anovulatory cycles and estrogen (although perhaps low) still dominates. (Chapter 8 provides details on this topic.)

Despite estrogen's reputation as a potential promoter of some kinds of cancer, it is believed to help prevent other kinds of cancer, such as colorectal cancer—possibly as a result of its action on blood lipids. Recent trials found that postmenopausal women using estrogen experience a 20 percent lower risk of developing colon cancer than women who have never taken the hormone. The effect of estrogen in preventing colon cancer has been studied over and over, and this study confirms the protective benefit.

Breast cancer

Some studies have found a relationship between breast cancer and estrogen use; others have found no such relationship. The topic is still under study after decades. A paradoxical finding comes from eight studies that compared women who had never used hormone-replacement therapy with those who were at the time they were diagnosed. Each study showed a lower chance of death for women who were receiving HRT at the time of their cancer diagnosis. In a recent nurses' health study conducted by the Hormone Foundation of Bethesda, Maryland, all women who received estrogens lived longer, with survival improving about 50 percent.

One possible explanation for the puzzling results is that estrogen may have stimulated tumor growth, allowing cancer to be diagnosed sooner than it would have been otherwise. Another potential explanation is that the tumors began to get smaller when estrogen therapy was halted. The increased medical attention that women who are on HRT receive is another potential explanation.

Bright Idea
The Cancer
Information
Service can
address your
questions about
the quality of
mammogram
facilities, about
how to find one,
and about
mammograms in
general. For
information, call
1-800-4-CANCER.

If one good thing can be said about estrogen supplementation's role in breast cancer, it's that tumors in women who are taking HRT don't seem to be as aggressive as tumors in women who aren't taking HRT. However, every woman should be aware that *there are real risks with HRT.*

A 1996 study by the Danish Cancer Society found that breast-cancer risk increases when women have been using hormones for five years or more and that the risk stays high as long as hormones are administered. Ten years or more on hormone therapy is associated with a 30 percent to 80 percent elevation of risk.

When women in the Danish study stopped HRT, however, their risk dropped two to five years later. The study did not distinguish a difference in risk with different types of estrogens. Moreover, adding progestins to an estrogen-replacement regimen didn't lower the risk. According to the results of that study, which appeared in the journal *Maturitas,* short-term HRT (less than five years) seemed to be safe as far as breast-cancer risk is concerned, but longer-term use led to a small but significant increase in risk.

Another study—this one done at the Instituto Nazionale Tumori in Milan, Italy—noted that high levels of androgens are linked with breast cancer. High serum-testosterone levels were found to precede the occurrence of breast cancer. And as we mentioned a bit earlier, it's recently been suggested that progestins, while used to treat some breast cancers, *could possibly* also in certain cases increase women's chances of developing breast cancer.

Endometrial cancer

Studies show that women run an increased risk of developing endometrial cancer (cancer of the uterine lining) when they take estrogen and do not take a progestin with it. But adding a progestin to estrogen-replacement therapy is believed to reduce that extra risk of endometrial cancer.

A 22-year retrospective study of women 45 and older estimated the yearly incidence of endometrial cancer among participants in a health plan and compared it with data on hormone-replacement therapy. In a March 1998 article in the journal *Gynecologic Oncology,* researchers Dr. Harry Ziel, Dr. William Finkle, and Dr. Sander Greenland reported that the lowest incidence of endometrial cancer (1991 through 1993) coincided with the highest estrogen prescriptions. That finding seems to contradict the general assumption that estrogen use increases the risk of endometrial cancer, but the researchers noted that use of progestins increased during the same time frame. Other studies confirm the likelihood of a protective effect through the addition of a progestin to hormone-replacement regimens.

Estrogen against osteoporosis?

Estrogen therapy for the prevention of osteoporosis is a controversial issue, but back in 1984, a National Institutes of Health group that was studying menopause felt strongly enough about the protective data to issue these recommendations:

- Cyclic estrogen therapy for women whose ovaries are removed before age 50 (in whom there are no medical reasons why it should not be given)

- Consider cyclic estrogen therapy for women who have gone through natural menopause (if they don't have contraindications and if they understand the risks involved and agree to regular medical evaluations)

Because the NIH data was based almost entirely on studies of white women, the recommendations pertained specifically to that group. For other ethnicities, determination on a case-by-case basis was suggested.

Watch Out!
Getting back lost bone isn't easy. Studies showing that estrogen reduces the continuing loss of bone also show that it doesn't restore the density of bones to premenopause levels.

In some studies, estrogen replacement was found to reduce the amount of bone loss and thereby slow or halt bone weakening. The number of hip and wrist fractures was reduced in women who started taking estrogen within the first few years after they went into menopause. The NIH panel, however, found no convincing evidence that estrogen therapy in elderly women actually prevented osteoporosis.

The extent to which estrogen helps curb osteoporosis is among the major reasons why physicians suggest it to their patients. But as you learn in upcoming pages, estrogen therapy carries significant risks, and women can take other measures to curb the rate of bone loss. If you're unsure whether you should consider estrogen-replacement therapy, talk it over with your physician. Two tests that are useful in assessing an individual's bone status are:

- DEXA scan—This test determines the density of bones in body sites that are most prone to fracture due to osteoporosis. The test can provide a baseline so comparisons can be made to women with peak bone mass as well as to women in an age-matched peer group.

- NTx (marketed as Osteomark)—This urine test measures the amount of bone breakdown products, called N-telopeptides, that are excreted in the urine. Because the substances are unique to bone, this is a good way to assess the amount of bone loss at a particular moment. It is also helpful in assessing whether or not medication is effective. If a repeat test done 2 to 3 months after therapy is started shows a 30 percent decline in this urinary bone marker, treatment can be considered effective.

Hormones and heart disease

A limited amount of data is available on the long-term safety of estrogen-progestin hormone replacement in postmenopausal women, but reports on early high-dose birth-control pills suggested a link between the oral contraceptives and a higher risk of heart attack and stroke. Early birth-control pills (those used in the 1960s) provided an estrogen dose nearly five times the dosages that are prescribed today.

Studies indicate that smoking and high blood pressure greatly increase the heart-attack risk of women who take the Pill (and of heart attacks at any age!). Increasing age seems to play a role as well. But reduced risk of coronary heart disease and stroke is associated with the use of estrogen-replacement therapy in postmenopausal women. Some studies suggest that estrogen therapy can reduce the risk of heart disease among women by as much as 50 percent. One criticism of these studies is that the women who took hormones tended to be more health conscious and physically active than the control group. This issue is currently under investigation in several studies that will be completed over the next few years. (In other studies, the reduced risk ranges from 25 percent to 80 percent.) Further research is being done on the role of female sex hormones in preventing or increasing the risk of heart disease.

Timesaver
To find out more about your risk of heart disease and stroke, visit the American Heart Association's Web site (www. americanheart.org).

Bright Idea
Dr. Nananda Francette Col's excellent book, *A Woman Doctor's Guide to Hormone Therapy* can help you determine whether or not taking HRT will increase or decrease your life expectancy. Using recent research on the potential risks and benefits of HRT, Dr. Col has generated easy to use charts and graphs that you use to objectively assess your own situation.

Estrogen and Alzheimer's disease

Women's increasing life spans put them at greater risk than men for developing Alzheimer's disease. As described in Chapter 6, estrogen seems to have a marked protective effect against Alzheimer's.

Researchers have found that postmenopausal women who receive estrogen are 40 percent to 60 percent less likely to develop Alzheimer's. After menopause, women who receive hormone-replacement therapy are about half as likely to develop Alzheimer's as women who do not receive HRT. In addition, the HRT group scored higher on standard mental-function tests than women who did not receive HRT. Multiple studies suggest that estrogen supplementation in postmenopausal women can protect them from getting Alzheimer's or at least stave off the onset of the disease.

The first controlled study of estrogen in Alzheimer's disease was conducted by Dr. Sanjay Asthana and colleagues at the U.S. Department of Veterans Affairs and the University of Washington, and reported in 1996. It involved six female Alzheimer's patients who were given estrogen supplementation for two months and six women who were given a placebo. Those in the estrogen group showed improved memory and attention (although the benefit diminished after estrogen therapy was stopped). Those in the placebo group didn't show significant changes.

Much to learn about HRT

The more scientists discover about sex hormones, the more complex the workings of those hormones in the body seem to be. As you see in this chapter, the results of some studies on major-disease risk differ in terms of when hormones can help and when they may hurt.

The science and art of hormone-replacement therapy is still developing, and if you're considering HRT, bear this fact in mind. Keep an eye on new information as it becomes available. Inform yourself about the options, benefits, and risks. Keep a line of communication open with a physician who is well versed in HRT. And talk with other women who are using HRT to see what *they* experience.

It's increasingly apparent that individual bio-chemistry can be delicate with regard to replacement therapy. Even slight variations in dosage, chemical structure, or even delivery system (such as creams vs. pills) can make for sizable differences in results. Chapter 8 delves into this issue.

Just the facts

- Estrogen is the most commonly prescribed hormone in the world.

- Surveys suggest that most women who begin hormone-replacement therapy don't stick with it long because of bleeding problems, cancer fears, weight gain, and failure of HRT to treat their symptoms.

- Progestins are typically prescribed along with estrogen in HRT to prevent pre-malignant changes in the uterus.

- Estrogen provides major protective effects against osteoporosis and cardiovascular disease.

Unofficially...
Health experts advise more studies on the dosage and duration of estrogen therapy in preventing, delaying, or alleviating Alzheimer's disease.

GET THE SCOOP ON...
Delivery systems ▪ Natural hormone-replacement
therapy ▪ Estrogens vs. progestins ▪
Over-the-counter remedies

Traditional or Natural: What Flavor of HRT?

Chapter 8

Deciding to give hormone-replacement therapy a try? Now you have a host of other decisions to make with your doctor. Should you supplement estrogen and a progestin together? Should you go for a pill, a cream, or a patch? What about all that you may have heard about natural progesterone and natural estrogen? Should you try an over-the-counter hormone supplement first?

Different *kinds* of hormone replacement tend to produce different *results*. Physicians have their methods of choice, including some options that weren't available 10 or even 5 years ago. But some women who don't find relief from the most popular kinds of HRT do find relief with new approaches. An open dialogue with your physician can help you explore what's going to work best for *you*.

This chapter discusses the effects of different patterns of hormone replacement, sorts out the issues of natural hormone replacement in comparison with conventional therapies, introduces the methods of hormone administration, and provides a word to the wise on over-the-counter hormone supplements.

Where do they get hormones from?

Although estrogen and progesterone were first isolated in the laboratory during the second and third decades of the 20th century, much remained to be learned about the effects of these hormones as supplemented in the human body.

Before scientists learned to synthesize hormones from plants, the chief sources of sex hormones were the sex glands of animals. Progesterone, for example, usually was obtained from the ovaries of sows or whales. During the 1930s, when the human placenta was found to be a rich source of progesterone, many placentas were harvested after childbirth, and progesterone was extracted for experimental use. The cost was high—around $80 per gram for early progesterone extracts. This high cost was undoubtedly a hindrance to widespread use of hormonal therapy.

Then a prodigious source of estrogen was found in, of all things, horse urine. The most typically prescribed estrogen in the United States today is Premarin, which consists of conjugated equine estrogens.)

But since Premarin was developed and synthetic progestins were patented, scientists have figured out how to derive both estrogens and progesterone from plant sources.

Russell Marker, an organic chemist in Pennsylvania, was fascinated by steroid hormones, and between the 1930s and '40s, he focused on plant steroids as a potential source of sex hormones. During the course of his investigations, Marker looked at the sarsaparilla family.

You may think of sarsaparilla as being what grannies in old Westerns drank at the local saloon, and indeed, it is still a soft drink today. The American Indians used it as a restorative centuries ago. During the 1600s, the Spanish brought the sarsaparilla plant (which is native to Mexico and Peru) from the New World to Europe, where men used it as a tonic for sexual potency.

Marker figured out how to turn a sapogenin, a plant steroid found in sarsaparilla, into a compound similar to progesterone. During one of his jungle expeditions for the sarsaparilla plant, Marker discovered that a species of wild yam can readily be processed to produce progesterone. When his methods were put into production, the price of progesterone dropped from $80 a gram to about 50 cents.

In 1944, Marker and his associates in Mexico opened a pharmaceutical-supply house called Syntex, providing Mexican wild yam–derived progesterone to meet the growing demand for progesterone in the treatment of menstrual difficulties. But with the science of the time, creating a dose large enough to be effective was a problem. A chemist with Marker's firm tinkered with things and came up with the first oral progestin, patented by Syntex and dubbed *norethindrone*. Eventually these synthetic oral progestins were combined with synthetic estrogens, and the first oral contraceptive pills were put on the market in 1960.

Cooking up a batch of hormones

The Mexican wild yams used to manufacture hormones are no relation to typical supermarket yams, and the human body is not thought to be able to synthesize progesterone or estrogen directly from

Unofficially...
The word *sarsaparilla* is derived from the Spanish words *zarza* (bramble) and *parilla* (little vine). The plants belong to the lily family. Sarsaparilla is not only a source for steroid hormones but also a flavoring agent in soft drinks, medicines, and other products.

Note! ➜
It is helpful to understand the terminology of hormones:

Progesterone: This is the hormone naturally found in the human body. If formed in the lab, it has a structure *identical* to that found in the body.

Progestin: This is a synthetically derived hormone with progesterone properties. The structure is similar but different from progesterone.

Progestogen: This is a substance that has progestational activity. It includes both progesterone and progestins.

wild yams. In the processing of this natural product, whole tubers of wild yams are typically mashed, fermented for a couple of days, dried in the sun, and hydrolyzed with mineral acid. Then a byproduct called *diosgenin* is extracted through the use of a solvent (such as light petroleum or heptane) that doesn't mix with water. Hormones are synthesized from the diosgenin, which is a plant steroid.

Progesterone can also be synthesized from soybeans and other vegetables. In fact, popular brands of hormones used in HRT come from some of the same places as natural progesterone. Estrogen, for example, can originate from a variety of sources, ranging from the equine estrogens in Premarin to beets, yams, soybeans, sweet potatoes, and other vegetable sources or totally synthetic preparations.

Pills, patches, creams, and choices

It used to be that when you took hormone-replacement therapy, you almost always took a pill. Now, however, a pill is just one of the following options:

- Oral forms (pills, capsules, sublingual lozenges (that is, absorbed from under the tongue), and liquids)
- Skin creams and gels
- Skin patches
- Vaginal creams and gels (used with an applicator)
- Vaginal rings
- Rectal suppositories

How do you take your estrogen?

In order to make sense of the advantages and disadvantages of the different routes by which hormones are administered, you need to understand where the medicines go once they enter your body.

- Medicine ingested in pill form is swallowed and absorbed by the stomach. Blood vessels surrounding the stomach absorb the medicine and then transport it *directly* to the liver where metabolism (breakdown) occurs. The immediate transportation of a medicine to the liver is called the "first pass effect," which essentially means the liver is exposed to a more intense dose of medicine in a relatively undiluted form. This mechanism is responsible for the liver's more dramatic response to medicine arriving via this route of administration as compared to other venues.

- Medicine administered transdermally (through the skin), sublingually (through the mucus membranes under the tongue), vaginally, and rectally is handled by the body in a different way. In these cases, medicine gets absorbed through small blood vessels (capillaries) near the administration site, and from there it feeds into the body's large blood vessels which eventually bring it to the liver. In this way the liver is not exposed to as dramatic a dose as in the oral route. This softens the impact on the liver, which can be good (decreased risk of gallstones and clots) or bad (less favorable cholesterol effect).

Thus you can see that medicines generally have the most impact on the site that gets first exposure. When vaginal hormones are administered, the vagina gets the bulk of the benefit, although high systemic levels can certainly be achieved via this route. In a similar way, women using transdermal estrogen preparations are advised to apply patches to the *lower* abdomen and hips rather than to the

Moneysaver
Many hormone types used in HRT are available as lower-cost generics, although the U.S. Food and Drug Administration has not yet granted approval for a generic equivalent of the most popularly prescribed estrogen, Premarin.

Bright Idea
Using a route of administration such as the transdermal patch allows medicine to bypass the stomach, thus eliminating side effects of nausea and vomiting for most women.

breast region in order to minimize intense exposure of hormones to the breasts.

The two main ways in which American women take estrogen are by pill (specifically, Premarin, which contains conjugated equine estrogens) and by patch or cream (specifically, estradiol, the main estrogen that the female body produces before menopause). But such *transdermal* (through the skin) systems as the patch and creams make for different metabolism in the body than pills do. Women who experience nausea when they take oral forms of estrogen may find that a patch or cream eliminates the problem.

Compared with oral forms of replacement therapy, estrogen patches deliver estrogens (usually, estradiol) in a more continuous manner, which tends to result in blood levels of estrone and estradiol that are closer to the levels that the body makes. One advantage of transdermal estrogen delivery is that it bypasses the digestive system and the liver, where metabolism of estrogen may lead to elevated blood pressure or other problems, such as increased formation of gallstones. When estrogen is taken orally, more of it arrives at the liver for processing than would normally be delivered by the ovaries (in the pre-menopausal state) through blood circulation.

Estrogen arriving at the liver in larger-than-physiologic dosages could have benefits as well as drawbacks. Because estrogen is associated with cardiovascular protection, one of the most heralded effects of oral forms is its capability to increase HDL cholesterol (known as the good type). HDL cholesterol is produced in the liver. When estrogen is metabolized in the liver, estrogen stimulates it to produce increased amounts of HDL cholesterol. Estrogen has another effect on the liver in that it stimulates the production of a protein, sex hormone binding globulin (SHBG), which functions in transporting hormones throughout the body in their inactive forms. This increase in (SHBG) proteins that bind to estrogen as well as to testosterone ultimately leaves less free-form active testosterone in the system.

Because oral estrogen can increase clotting potential (another liver metabolism effect), women who are subject to blood clots may be well advised to think about other forms, of hormone delivery, such as transdermal forms that bypass direct metabolization in the liver. Sometimes direct metabolism in the liver induces high blood pressure via an intricate network of hormone regulators in the body. Note that the majority of women taking oral HRT do *not* develop high blood pressure, although this reaction does sometimes occur and should be monitored.

Results of a 1994 study reported by the Mayo Clinic suggest that at least theoretically, transdermal estrogen therapy may be more beneficial than oral estrogen therapy for women who smoke cigarettes, have migraine headaches, high triglyceride levels, liver disorders, fibrocystic breast disease, or a history of thromboembolism (blood clots).

But, the study noted, women who have high cholesterol may respond better to an orally administered estrogen. High cholesterol may be balanced by the production of good cholesterol, thanks to orally administered estrogen.

Transdermal patches have been shown to produce favorable lipid profiles, prevent loss of bone, relieve hot flashes, and prevent vaginal atrophy, just

Watch Out!
About 15 percent of women using estrogen patches, such as Estraderm, have some localized skin irritation, but most don't stop therapy because of it. When using a patch, remove the protective backing and allow the patch to "breathe" for a minute prior to applying it to the skin. This allows alcohol to evaporate and decreases the risk of skin irritation. Sometimes, humid, hot weather interferes with how the patches adhere to the skin.

as oral hormones do. Even though the lipid benefits are not quite as dramatic with transdermal administration, estrogen by itself is such a powerful agent, that the overall effect is an improvement in cholesterol ratios and a decrease in triglycerides. The transdermal patch has several advantages over pills. It may be more convenient for women who dislike or forget to take pills. Instead of daily administration it requires application once or twice a week, depending on the brand. For those women who get nauseated by oral HRT it literally bypasses this problem by circumventing the stomach! Patches also come in different strengths, so dosages can be adjusted—the higher the dose, the larger the patch.

The transdermal patch has a design that allows slow, steady, release of hormones from the patch into the skin. The patch has a pliable backing that prevents the hormone from being rubbed off or absorbed onto clothing. This is an important benefit since it ensures reliable delivery of the medicine and prevents it from being transferred during intimate contact to a sexual partner. This type of absorption can occur for example with creams applied to the skin or vagina. Sex partners have occasionally noted breast tenderness when inadvertently exposed to these hormones.

Natural transdermal creams and gels have become more popular recently. Unlike the patch, there is less precision in terms of dosing, daily administration is required, and sex partners may be exposed to potent medication.

Estrogen-replacement therapy can also be delivered vaginally. When given in this fashion the main objective is usually relief of urogenital atrophy. Urogenital atrophy refers to thinning and loss of tone of the vagina and bladder. Because the bladder

Bright Idea
In the past, transdermal patches only supplied estrogen. This meant women with a uterus in place had to take an oral progestational agent along with the patch. The recent introduction of new a transdermal system that supplies both estrogen and a progestin (CombiPatch) now permits women to get total HRT via the transdermal route.

is located adjacent to the vagina, it is also nourished by estrogen. The changes that occur in the vagina and the bladder with menopausal decreases in estrogen are often dramatic. Intercourse may become painful (the medical term for this pain is dyspareunia) due to decreased lubrication, thinning of the vaginal walls, and shrinking of vaginal caliber. The normal bacterial composition of the vagina often changes along with the decrease in estrogen. The vagina normally has a composition of bacteria which is called "the vaginal flora." It is this composition of bacteria that are responsible for the vagina's ability to maintain its characteristic odor, to keep its lining healthy, and to prevent its overgrowth with less favorable bacteria and yeast. When the normal vaginal flora is disrupted, imbalance may occur, leading to infection or irritation. The most protective vaginal bacteria are the lactobacillus bacteria, the bacteria found in yogurt. When estrogen decreases during menopause, the vaginal flora changes and lactobacillus levels decrease. The changes in bacterial composition along with physical changes such as vaginal thinning make the vagina more susceptible to irritation and infection. When estrogen is replaced these changes can be reversed; vaginal infection rates decrease and painful intercourse declines. (See Chapter 12 for more information on this problem).

The bladder also undergoes changes during menopause because it is the vagina's next door neighbor, sharing a common wall just like two apartments do in an apartment building. Loss of estrogen causes the bladder walls to thin and weaken. Many women find bladder symptoms that were manageable prior to menopause become worse with menopause. Urinary incontinence, which is the involuntary loss of urine, is often the result of two common causes:

- **Urinary stress incontinence (USI).** This is a loss of bladder control due to structural changes in the bladder, such as the loss of support in the urethra, the tube that runs from the bladder to the vulva. Often, laughing or coughing results in loss of urine. While most women experience these losses from time to time, women with USI frequently wet themselves with even minor changes in activity.

- **Urge incontinence (also called detrussor instability).** This is a loss of bladder control due to uninhibited bladder contractions. With urge incontinence there is a sudden overwhelming urge to urinate that cannot be controlled, resulting in inappropriate wetting.

There can be other, less common causes of incontinence, such as neurological disorders (multiple sclerosis, Parkinson's disease, stroke, spinal cord damage); diabetes; decreased bladder capacity due to radiation damage; and extrinsic compression due to fibroids.

The evaluation of incontinence starts with a detailed history of symptoms followed by a careful pelvic and urologic exam. Cystometrics, a test that measures the bladder's ability to fill and empty, is often critical in arriving at the proper diagnosis. Many times urge and stress incontinence coexist to varying degrees. Cystometrics can determine the extent that each plays in incontinence. With this knowledge, treatment can be given in a rational manner.

Stress incontinence can be treated with pelvic strengthening exercises (which helps in mild cases) or with pelvic reconstructive surgery. Urge incontinence is treated with behavior modification (increasing the frequency of voiding) or with medications. New medications (Detrol and Ditropan XL) recently put on the market have fewer side effects (dry mouth, constipation, urinary retention, blurred vision) than earlier medications. These medications inhibit bladder contractions thereby decreasing urgency and bladder accidents. See Chapter 9 for more about specific incontinence medications.

While the treatment for both types of incontinence is different, postmenopausal women treated with HRT or with vaginal estrogen alone often find improvement. Addition of estrogen is often the first step in treating incontinence, and women with mild problems often benefit. Estrogen increases blood flow to the vagina and bladder and this helps restore bladder tone and health.

Estrogen is readily absorbed through the vaginal lining and if given in large amounts, blood levels comparable to those from the oral route are reached. Women using this vaginal treatment for urogenital atrophy must not use large doses. When given in small amounts (1 gram of Premarin cream per week, for example), the vagina can be nourished without exposing the rest of the body to high estrogen levels. For those women who are suffering from urogenital atrophy and don't desire or need full HRT, vaginal estrogen therapy is ideal. When given in small amounts, endometrial hyperplasia and breast cancer risk is not increased.

Vaginal estrogen can be given in the following ways: via creams or via a vaginal ring (Estring). The vaginal ring is a newly introduced method that has a very soft, pliable silastic (silicone) ring that is easily inserted into the vagina. It releases a minimal continuous dose of estradiol directly to the vagina over a three-month interval. Once a woman is instructed on its insertion, she can easily replace it herself every three months. Side effects are minimal. Sometimes increased vaginal discharge occurs. One advantage is that it delivers a controlled, small dose of hormone and bypasses the risk of overexposure.

Table 8.1 describes the advantages and drawbacks of different methods of estrogen administration.

The recently introduced vaginal ring isn't the last word in hormone-delivery options. The companies that provide hormones, as well as academic researchers and physicians, are continuing to look for the best ways to administer them. Among the new methods being developed is an IUD (intrauterine device) that releases a stream of hormones. Early research on progestin-releasing IUDs suggests that although increased spotting occurs compared with other methods, the IUDs may be an effective and safe way to balance endometrial exposure to estrogen in postmenopausal women.

What brand names are you likely to see on your doctor's prescription pad? Following are some of the popular estrogen brands and formulations, listed by how you take them:

Unofficially...
A compounding pharmacy is a pharmacy with the capability to make prescriptions to a doctor's specifications, using generic medicines. These pharmacies are able to produce cream, ointment, or capsule combinations on-site.

Pills

Bi-Est: estriol and estradiol; from a compounding pharmacy

Estrace: estradiol

Estradiol: estradiol

Estratab esterified estrogens (mixture of estrogenic substances, but principally estrone)

Estriol: estriol

TABLE 8.1: CHARACTERISTICS OF ESTROGEN-ADMINISTRATION METHODS

Method	Advantages	Drawbacks
Oral (pills, liquids, capsules, and so on.)	Pills have been extensively tested; oral forms are well tolerated by most women; oral forms may be less expensive and beneficial for women with high cholesterol.	Other forms of HRT should be considered for women who smoke or who tend to develop gallstones, blood clots, migraines, high triglycerides, fibrocystic breast disease, or liver disease. May cause nausea.
Oral (sublingual lozenges)	Some hormone is absorbed via mucous membranes in your mouth rather than passing through digestive system.	Administration more involved than swallowing pills

Bypasses liver |
| Patches | Continuous release of hormone; bypass liver. Don't require daily dosing. | May cause skin irritation in some women; may have adherence problems in hot, humid weather. |
| Skin creams and gels | Bypass liver; deliver more doses than pills | |
| Vaginal creams and gels | Bypass liver; tend to target specific tissues

Most prominent effect to vagina; little systemic effect. | May be messy, with cream leaking out on underwear. Take care not to expose sex partners. |
| Vaginal rings | Target specific tissues; bypass liver | Potential vaginal irritation and infection |
| Rectal suppositories | Bypass liver | Application may be annoying. |

Note: Methods of administration can be combined when you're adding a progesterone to the regimen, such as using an estrogen patch but oral form of progestin.

Estrone: estrone

Menest: esterified estrogens

Ogen: estropipate; a form of estrone

Ortho-Est: estropipate

Premarin: conjugated equine estrogens (CEE)

Tri-Est: estriol, estradiol, and estrone; a combination of these three estrogens prepared by a compounding pharmacy usually in the following proportions: estriol 80 percent, estradiol 10 percent, estrone 10 percent.

Note! ➡
Most oral HRT is administered in pill form, but sublingual lozenges, capsules, liquids, and other forms can be provided by a compounding pharmacy, according to your doctor's prescription.

Patches

Alora: estradiol

Climara: estradiol

Esclim: estradiol

Estraderm: estradiol

Estradiol: estradiol

FemPatch: estradiol

Vivelle: estradiol

Vaginal creams

Estrace: estradiol

Estradiol: estradiol

Estriol: estriol

Estrone: estrone

Ogen: estropipate; a form of estrone

Premarin: conjugated equine estrogens (CEE)

Vaginal rings

Estring: estradiol (used for three months)

Skin creams

Bi-Est: 80 percent estriol, 20 percent estradiol

Estradiol: estradiol

Estriol: estriol

Estrone: estrone

Tri-Est: 80 percent estriol, 10 percent estrone,
     10 percent estradiol

Other estrogen blends can be made by *compounding pharmacies,* where Bi-Est and Tri-Est are formulated. In addition, combinations of estrogens, progesterone, and testosterone can be formulated in capsules and creams.

Providing progesterone and progestins

Like estrogen, progesterone and progestins can be administered in different ways. Progestins are typically given in pill form, but they're available in other forms, such as vaginal gels. Natural progesterone, which has to be compounded by a full-service pharmacy that has the equipment to do so, can be provided in oral forms (capsules, pills, liquids, sublinguals, and so on) and is often provided for transdermal use as a cream or gel. Vaginal creams or gels can also be formulated, as can rectal suppositories. Progesterone and progestins are metabolized by the liver in the same manner as estrogen. Studies show progesterone and progestins lower HDL, the good cholesterol, but do not negate estrogen's overall beneficial effects on the heart. More research is under way to evaluate which forms have the most impact. Preliminary results imply progesterone may have more favorable effects on the heart than progestins.

New forms of progesterone are now available from the pharmaceutical companies in oral and vaginal forms. They are just beginning to be marketed for HRT use, such as Solvay Pharmaceuticals, Inc.'s Prometrium (progesterone, USP). Capsules were FDA approved for use in HRT in late

1998. Progestin injections have been used for contraception as well as for non-menopausal diseases such as endometriosis (a disease characterized by abnormally located endometrial lining). At the present time their use in HRT does not appear to be imminent.

One big problem with oral delivery of progestins or progesterone is the fact that so much has to be supplied in order to have an effect. But micronization of progesterone (which means breaking it into tiny, easily absorbed particles) seems to enhance absorption. Early studies show that micronized progesterone is readily absorbed when administered orally.

Following are popular progestin and progesterone brands, listed by their method of administration:

Pills

Amen: medroxyprogesterone acetate

Aygestin: norethindrone acetate

Curretab: medroxyprogesterone acetate

Cycrin: medroxyprogesterone acetate

Medroxyprogesterone acetate: generic form

Norlutate: norethindrone acetate

Progesterone: natural micronized progesterone; from a compounding pharmacy

Prometrium: progesterone, USP; capsules; oral micronized progesterone

Provera: medroxyprogesterone acetate

Progesterone creams, gels, and suppositories

Crinone (vaginal gel): micronized progesterone

Note! →
Like estrogen, progestins in pill form may provide higher-than-normal physiologic dosages due to the body's metabolism of the hormone. A large dose is required for an effective amount to remain for use by the body.

Progesterone (gel, cream, or vaginal and rectal sup-
     pository): micronized natural progesterone;
     from compounding pharmacy

Skin creams and gels have become popular,
particularly for the administration of natural progesterone. Because the body's premenopausal manufacture of sex hormones takes place largely in and
around female reproductive organs, in some cases,
it can be beneficial to target therapy toward those
tissues rather than seek high systemic levels of a hormone whose actions elsewhere in the body may be
unwanted. Vaginally delivered hormones (creams,
gels, and suppositories) work toward that end. If
you don't tolerate progestins or progesterone well
through other delivery methods, you may want to
discuss targeted delivery with your doctor.

Physicians sometimes give injections of progestins to control unusual and heavy uterine bleeding or the opposite: a lack of menstruation, known
as *amenorrhea*. Injected progestins are also used in
the treatment of kidney and uterine cancer, and as
a birth-control measure (Depo-Provera, for example). Injections are not commonly used in *routine*
HRT.

Scientists have been studying the possible use for
HRT of intrauterine devices (IUDs), like those that
have been used in contraception. Researchers hope
that IUDs that supply progesterone or a progestin
(such as Progestasert) may be useful in reducing
endometrial hyperplasia in postmenopausal women
who are on estrogen therapy, without the systemic
effects of progesterone and progestins, such as
bloating.

An intrauterine device used for HRT can
be expected to carry drawbacks similar to those of

conventional IUDs, such as the chance of spotting or bleeding, discomfort on insertion, and a small risk of uterine perforation during insertion. A disadvantage of the current Progestasert IUD is its need for yearly replacement—besides being costly, insertion of this device can sometimes be uncomfortable.

A 1995 Finnish study found that an IUD supplying the progestin levonorgestrel resulted in few side effects, except for some abdominal cramps and spotting during the early months of use.

Combinations

In the interest of making HRT easier to take, some combination products have been formulated: estrogen and progestins—and sometimes estrogen with testosterone. Following are some popular brands:

Estrogen/progestin (oral)

PremPro: conjugated estrogens and medroxyprogesterone acetate

PremPhase: conjugated estrogens and medroxyprogesterone acetate

Estrogen/Progestin (patch)

CombiPatch: estradiol and norethindrone acetate

Estrogen/testosterone (oral)

Estratest: esterified estrogens and methyltestosterone

Estratest HS: esterified estrogens and methyltestosterone (the half strength version of Estratest)

Which estrogen? which progestin?

Decided to pack a patch, tote a pill case, or give the ring a try? Your job's not over. Different methods of delivering hormones to your body differ in effect, and the *type* of hormone that you take can make a difference as well. In other words, all estrogens are not alike, and neither are all progestins (which are not the same thing as progesterone).

Estrogens

Estradiol (E2), the estrogen that your ovaries produce when you're fertile, is the most abundant estrogen in your body. The weaker estrogen estrone (E1), which is made from estradiol, is the kind that predominates in your body after menopause because it is made in other locations in your body (including fat cells). Estriol (E3), which is frequently prescribed in Europe, is the third human estrogen—a weak one that your body makes (from estradiol) in massive quantities when you're pregnant. Resear-chers believe that estriol may protect against certain cancers.

It should be noted that there have not been any well run studies supporting the claim that estriol has an anticancer effect. These claims are the result of small studies that showed estriol had an inhibitory effect on breast tumors in rats. These results have not been reproduced in human studies and to date it is still an unsubstantiated claim. When given in doses equal in strength estriol stimulates endometrial hyperplasia (a precancerous condition in the uterus) as does estradiol.

If you take a form of estrogen other than estrone orally, you may end up with estrone anyway because the body tends to metabolize orally administered estrogens into estrone. Table 8.3 lists some characteristics of different human estrogens.

Timesaver
Remember that some estrogens and progestins are typically available in a certain form— patch or vaginal ring, for example. If you're set on a certain form of delivery, that form may dictate the actual hormone that could wind up with a prescription for.

Note! ➡
Tri-Est, which provides all three estrogens, typically does so in a ratio of 80 percent estriol, 10 percent estradiol, and 10 percent estrone. Bi-Est, another popular combination contains 80 percent estriol and 20 percent estradiol. A compounding pharmacy, however, can make other combinations.

TABLE 8.3: MAIN HUMAN ESTROGENS

Estrogen	Description
Estradiol (E2)	Most abundant during fertile years
Estrone (E1)	Weak estrogen; other estrogens administered orally tend to be metabolized into estrone
Estriol (E3)	May have anticancer characteristics; can cause nausea in high doses

The most commonly prescribed estrogen, Premarin, is not actually a synthetic, but a combination of estrogens that naturally occur in horses. Premarin is, however, nearly half estrone (which *is* natural to human females). Several million women take Premarin, which has been widely studied for safety and efficacy.

The side effects associated with Premarin resemble those of a wide range of estrogens on the market: appetite loss, nausea, diarrhea, swollen feet and ankles, breast swelling and discomfort, acne, and so on. Abdominal cramps and abnormal vaginal bleeding can also be associated with estrogen use, and estrogen may increase the risk of blood clots.

Multiple studies have shown a Premarin dose of 0.625 to be most beneficial to maintaining bone density. Equivalent doses of estradiol are believed to have the same benefits, although definitive studies are currently underway. Some women find dosages of Premarin 0.625 (or the estradiol equivalent) inadequate in relieving hot flashes and other menopausal symptoms. Dosages can be increased, although the goal is to give the lowest dose effective in maintaining bone strength while concomitantly relieving menopause symptoms.

Progestins

Progestins—those chemically similar cousins of progesterone—are used not only in HRT, to help balance the effects of estrogen, but also in birth-control pills and for treatment of abnormal uterine bleeding. Progestins are also used to treat the *lack* of regular periods (amenorrhea). Some progestins, such as megestrol acetate (Megace), are used to treat women who have had cancer of the uterus or breast.

Among the unwanted side effects of progestins is the suppression of HDL cholesterol—the so-called good cholesterol, which helps balance the amount of LDL (the so-called bad cholesterol) in our systems. Some progestins behave androgenically (that is, behaving like a male hormone), producing unwanted male-hormone effects such as acne, loss of scalp hair, or a slight increase in the amount or thickness of body hair. Others can have more effects along the lines of estrogen, acting as antiandrogens (that is, antagonizing male hormone effects) by improving the complexion or decreasing unwanted growth of body hair.

Successful HRT is an issue of balance, and a progestin that causes unwanted side effects in one woman may be the right prescription for another woman.

Progestins can typically be divided into two categories: 19-nor-testosterone derivatives (such as norethindrone) and norgestrel and C-21 progestins (such as medroxyprogesterone acetate). The more-androgenic progestins often have *nor* in their names, but not all *nor* progestins are necessarily particularly androgenic.

"Equivalent dose" is a term used to describe the dosage of one compound that has an equal biological effect as another similar compound. If you are taking traditional HRT and want to change to natural HRT equivalent dosing will enable you to make an easy transition. The following estrogens have equivalent doses: Premarin 0.625 milligrams;

Oral estradiol 1.0 milligram;

Transdermal estradiol .05 milligrams.

Among the progestins, norethindrone acetate (NETA), which is often used in birth-control pills, has a reputation for having more androgenic effects in some women's systems than medroxyprogesterone acetate does. If you have problems with acne or have other androgenic effects, you may want to consider a lower dose of progestin or natural progesterone.

Elevated levels of male hormones can cause acne in certain women by increasing the secretion of sebum from sebaceous glands and sometimes causing follicles to harden, thereby exacerbating the problem. Birth-control pills are sometimes prescribed to help control acne in women.

You can easily see how skin problems can arise during perimenopause and menopause, when hormone levels are fluctuating. Low levels of estrogen (with the presence of androgens) can encourage skin problems. High levels of androgens stimulate the secretion of sebum, which is the oily substance that causes acne. In a woman who has balanced hormone levels, estrogen as it naturally occurs raises levels of sex-hormone-binding globulin (SHBG). The SHBG offsets the effect of the androgens because it binds with free-circulating testosterone and other male hormones, thereby reducing their levels and their effects.

A common side effect of systemic progestins is a change in the pattern of uterine bleeding. This potential for abnormal or annoying bleeding is the main reason women give for discontinuing HRT. For many years progestins were given in a sequential manner. Typically they were taken for 10 to 14 days of the month in order to offset estrogen's stimulatory effect to the uterus. Over time it was appreciated that lower doses of progestin offered

Watch Out!
Some progestins may be more androgenic than others. In many women, typical androgenicity problems include acne and oily skin. More masculinizing patterns, such as scalp-hair loss and a noticeable increase in body hair, usually do not occur with normal levels of HRT.

protection comparable to high doses. Research shows that *daily* use of 2.5 milligrams of medroxy-progesterone as part of HRT is a safe way to avoid uterine cancer. It is also a way to prevent bleeding entirely (amenorrhea), which makes it an attractive method to give hormones. Thus, combined HRT consisting of daily doses of estrogen plus a low dose of a progestin is a safe and attractive mode of giving hormones. Some women *never* achieve amenorrhea with continuous low dose progestin. These women ultimately find frequent staining and bleeding at unpredictable times very annoying. They tend to do better with cyclic use of progestin as mentioned above.

Not all progestins have the same side effects, however. The following list describes other side effects that sometimes occur with progestins:

- Abdominal cramps and pain
- Acne
- Breast pain or tenderness
- Brown spots on skin exposed to sunlight
- Changes in amount or texture of body and scalp hair
- Changes in uterine bleeding pattern
- Decreased libido
- Depression
- Edema
- Elevated-blood-sugar symptoms (dry mouth, frequent urination, reduced appetite, and increased thirst)
- Galactorrhea (unexpected breast milk production)
- Headaches

TimeSaver
Equivalent doses for progesterone and progestin medications are: Medroxyprogesterone 2.5 milligrams; Oral micronized prog-esterone 100 micrograms.

- Hot flashes

- Insomnia

- Mood changes

- Nausea

- Nervousness

- Rashes

- Tiredness

- Weakness

- Weight gain

Note! ➜
Promptly advise
your doctor if
you experience
any notable side
effects from HRT.

In high doses, some progestins have been associated with blood clots, heart attacks, strokes, liver disorders, and eye problems, although it's not certain whether progestins cause the problems or simply exacerbate existing conditions. Seek medical help immediately if you experience any of these rare side effects or symptoms that may indicate them, such as severe or sudden headache (which can indicate blood-clotting problems); shortness of breath without obvious cause; change in your speech, coordination, or vision; or numbness or pain in your chest or extremities.

Androgens

When androgens (such as testosterone) are added to HRT, patient and physician must watch for more-pronounced virilizing effects, such as increased growth of body hair. If you are low in testosterone, however, adding testosterone to your daily HRT regimen may help; some women say that it helps considerably with libido and energy. Balance is what's important.

Researchers have found that compared with estrogen therapy alone, estrogen-androgen therapy may not only enhance libido, energy, and sense of well-being, but also offer increased protection against osteoporosis. As Chapter 7 notes, however, the beneficial effect of estrogen on cholesterol may be partially offset by introducing androgens to HRT.

Natural hormone replacement

A growing undercurrent of opinion is leaning toward natural hormone-replacement therapy instead of replacement with traditional synthetic or animal-derived versions of estrogen and progestins. Proponents hold that they simply act differently in the human body than one's own hormones do—and that natural-hormone therapy may offer more promise and fewer problems.

On the other side of the coin, the kinds of estrogen and progestins that have been used for many years have the benefit of thorough testing, and millions of women find help through them. To be technical about it, the so-called natural estrogens and progesterone could be described as synthetics because they are synthesized from plant sources. The difference between natural progesterone and the progestins is in the structure of the molecules themselves.

The hullabaloo over natural progesterone

While estrogen has a reputation among many gynecologists as being the "happy hormone,"—natural progesterone has entered the limelight recently as a popular panacea for menopause problems. One of the chief proponents of natural progesterone is Dr. John R. Lee, M.D., who suggests that the root of many menopausal difficulties is not estrogen deficiency, but a relative lack of progesterone. The idea is detailed in Lee's book (with Virginia Hopkins)

What Your Doctor May Not Tell You About Menopause: The Breakthrough Book on Natural Progesterone.

Moneysaver
Over-the-counter natural-proges-terone creams tend to be as expensive as, or more expensive than, com-pounded natural progesterone prescribed by a physician.

When progesterone is severely deficient, Lee posits, even minimal amounts of estrogen in the system can set up an estrogen-dominance syndrome that can be responsible for problems from acceleration of the aging process to water retention and from breast tenderness to weight gain. Lee suggests that estrogen excess in the presence of progesterone deficiency (that is, estrogen dominance) is the root of most perimenopausal and menopausal problems. Many women find relief of menopausal symptoms when using progesterone creams, though Lee's work is controversial in the medical community, with critics citing a lack of research on progesterone-only supplementation in support of his views. More research is underway to investigate the merits of progesterone therapy, and pharmaceutical manufacturers are beginning to bring brand name progesterone to market for HRT use.

Mixed messages arriving at the cell are, Lee says, responsible for adverse reactions to progestins which are uncharacteristic of natural progesterone. Lee cites natural progesterone as leading to improved blood lipid profiles, as well as the normalization of libido and sleep patterns, and he suggests it enhances fertility and diminishes hirsutism while allowing regrowth of scalp hair. Lee also describes natural progesterone as protective against breast cancer.

There are certainly reports supporting the role of our own progesterone in ensuring health, such as the one described in chapter 4 wherein women with breast cancer fared much better after surgery completed during the progesterone-rich phase of their menstrual cycle than during the phase when it is largely absent. Mainstream medicine remains unconvinced that natural progesterone is a cure-all, but some physicians are turning their attention to the use of both naturally occurring progesterone and human estrogens, as consumer interest in natural HRT has burgeoned and as research progresses.

Progesterone or Progestin?

Since progestin molecules are not the same as the progesterone our bodies make, the door is left open for them to act in different ways than either our own progesterone or lab-manufactured progesterone, which is identical in molecular structure to human progesterone. More research should shed light on the benefits and drawbacks of supplementing either.

Some interesting studies have been conducted illustrating differences in responses to progestins versus progesterone. What is being learned may have an impact on cholesterol and heart disease considerations in HRT. In human studies more favorable HDL cholesterol levels have resulted from HRT regimens using progesterone than from those using the progestin medroxyprogesterone acetate. And data from a study in primates suggests progesterone could potentially be better than progestin in terms of cardiovascular health, when combined with an estrogen in HRT.

Testing of progesterone in HRT has typically included it in combination with estrogen. One such study is the extensive Postmenopausal Estrogen/Progestin Interventions (PEPI) Trial, a multicenter study sponsored in part by the National Institutes of Health. The trials involve 875 postmenopausal

Unofficially...
During pregnancy, the body's normal production of progesterone increases several hundred times.

Unofficially...
Synthetic progestins can be significantly more potent than natural progesterone—as much as 2,000 times more potent, in some cases.

Watch Out!
Natural proges-
terone can have
a calming effect
on the central
nervous system,
but at higher
dosages, it can
make you drowsy.

women aged 45 to 64 years. According to 1995 results, women who took conjugated estrogens and micronized progesterone experienced an average increase in HDL ("good cholesterol") levels close to three times the increase experienced by users of conjugated estrogens and the progestin medrox-yprogesterone acetate, giving it the most favorable HDL cholesterol outcome of the treatment options in that study.

A small, year-long study at Vanderbilt University Medical Center (Nashville, Tennessee) in 1989 compared groups of 5 menopausal women each who took either a combination of micronized estradiol and progesterone, or a combination of conjugated estrogens and the progestin medroxyprogesterone acetate. While both groups experienced an increase in the "good" HDL cholesterol, only the group taking estradiol and progesterone experienced a decrease in total cholesterol, and members also had less withdrawal bleeding than the other group.

The results of a 1997 study at the NIH-supported Oregon Regional Primate Research Center suggest that (at least in monkeys) a hormone replacement regimen including progesterone may be safer for the heart than a regimen including a commonly used progestin. Scientists studied a dozen rhesus monkeys whose ovaries had been removed to simulate menopause, and put them on HRT. One group received estrogen and progesterone while the other group received estrogen and medroxyprogesterone acetate. Then researchers induced coronary vasospasms (similar to those in heart attacks) in the monkeys, and measured how well or poorly recovery took place.

The animals that had received estrogen and progesterone experienced brief artery constrictions but were protected from deadly vasospasm—blood flow quickly went back to normal. But in the monkey group receiving medroxyprogesterone acetate, spasms were severe and coronary arteries remained constricted long enough to pose a threat to life (until a vasodilating agent was injected to reverse the effect). Researchers concluded medroxyprogesterone in contrast to progesterone increases the risk of coronary vasospasm.

These studies highlight a relatively new awareness of the potentially different behavior in HRT of supplementary progesterone versus progestins.

Natural hormones by prescription or over-the-counter

Natural hormone preparations can be made up by a compounding pharmacy in whatever dosage your doctor desires. The female body typically produces 20 to 24 milligrams of progesterone daily during the last 12 to 14 days of her menstrual cycle, and natural progesterone supplementation at physiologic levels mimics that dosage.

Although oral and other forms of natural progesterone are available, compounded creams are popular, well absorbed, and dosed as so many milligrams (usually 30 to 100) per gram of cream. A compounding pharmacy generally can supply an applicator for measuring out the correct dose, according to your physician's instructions. If you are to take 20 milligrams per day and are using a 10 percent cream, for example, you might use two daily doses of 10 milligrams each, rubbed into your palms and the fatty areas of your body. Micronized oral progesterone is usually given in doses of 100 milligrams per day for continuous dose regimens. For cyclic regimens a dose of 200 milligrams for 12 to 14

Unofficially...
During pregnancy, the body's normal production of progesterone increases by several hundred times.

days can be given. Unfortunately the body's ability to absorb oral progesterone can vary, which sometimes leads to annoying spotting. Sometimes this can be averted by taking the hormone in divided doses throughout the day, although many women find this annoying. Also, it must be emphasized that definitive studies on the risks and benefits of natural progesterone are pending.

Two natural progesterone products were recently introduced by pharmaceutical companies with the intention of being used to treat fertility and menstrual disorders. Prometrium is an oral form containing 100 milligrams of progesterone. It contains peanut oil (which enhances its absorption). If you are allergic to peanuts, do not take this product. Crinone vaginal gel is the other product. It comes in two strengths, 4 and 8 percent. The lower dose form has been used in Europe for HRT applied twice weekly for continuous therapy or every other day for six doses per month for cyclic therapy.

A growing market in over-the-counter natural progesterone (and natural estrogen) has arisen. Many low-dose products are available, but there is some concern about whether they actually contain progesterone or simply wild yam or other botanicals that the body cannot convert to progesterone. Some critics have called this the "wild yam scam" since the conversion to progesterone can only be done in a laboratory.

Some women report that wild yams and other natural foods and herbs give them the positive effects that they expect from natural progesterone (see Chapter 13 on herbs for menopause). To find an over-the-counter product that contains bioavailable natural progesterone, which means a form of

Watch Out!
Even over-the-counter progesterone preparations can alter your menstrual cycle. Cycling women are often advised to use progesterone creams only during the last half of their cycle (from ovulation on) and then to stop for a week to allow for normal menstruation.

progesterone that the body can use, look for the word *progesterone* among the ingredients.

The quantities of progesterone in different products can vary significantly, from less than 5 milligrams per ounce to more than 1,000 milligrams per ounce. Among the most widely available fairly high-concentration products are Feminique (manufactured by Country Life) and ProGest (Transitions for Health).

Emerita ProGest, for example, provides 450 milligrams of progesterone per ounce of cream, meaning that physiologic dosages range from ¼ to ½ teaspoon twice daily.

Just as over-the-counter progesterone creams are becoming widely available, over-the-counter phytoestrogen creams and vaginal gels are making increased appearances. The latter compounds usually contain herbs rather than specifically extracted estrogens. For more information on this topic, see Chapter 13.

Some of the prescription estrogens that are currently available are derived from plant sources, even if they're not frequently promoted as such. These estrogens include Climara (manufactured by Berlex, and made from yams and beets), Estrace (Mead Johnson; made from yams and soy), and Ogen (Upjohn; made from various vegetable sources).

Choices in HRT: Putting it all together

As you can see from this chapter, there are *plenty* of choices you and your doctor can make when choosing a regimen for HRT. Factors to consider include the following:

Route of administration: The most common choices include oral and transdermal administration. Those women with cardiovascular risk factors

Bright Idea
Some women report that they are better able to handle low-dosage progesterone creams (available either by prescription or over the counter), so consider starting conservatively and working toward balance.

Timesaver
Check labels for the phrase *U.S.P. Progesterone.* (*U.S.P.* stands for *United States Pharmacopoeia*). This phrase indicates a progesterone that exactly duplicates the progesterone that your body makes, to differentiate it from synthetic progestins.

will usually benefit from oral use whereas women with sensitive stomachs, clotting problems, gallstones, and migraine headaches may be better off with transdermal use. All routes appear to benefit the bones and vagina.

Continuous vs. cyclic administration: As mentioned earlier in this chapter continuous combined HRT gives the benefit of amenorrhea (no bleeding) along with ease of use—you simply take the same medicine each and every day. It is superior to cyclic regimens for those women with migraine headaches and sensitivity to hormone fluctuations (including moodiness, bloating, and breast tenderness.) These regimens contain very low doses of progestins, a plus for those sensitive to their side effects. When you start a continuous regimen be prepared for staining or bleeding at unpredictable times for the first three to six months of use. (If you did not have abnormal bleeding prior to HRT use, this is not worrisome, only annoying.) The bleeding will generally resolve over time, although 20 percent of women fail to attain amenorrhea for various reasons. Women with fibroids have more difficulties as do women who are newly menopausal (the body's own hormone levels may still be fluctuating, which results in more frequent bleeding). Those women who cannot tolerate continuous therapy as well as those women who prefer to continue to menstruate will generally do well on one of several cyclic regimens:

> Estrogen alone for 14 days/estrogen and progestagen for 14 days.
>
> Estrogen alone for 15 days/estrogen and progestagen for the next 10 days/no medicine for the rest of the month

Estrogen every day/add progestagen for 12 days of the month (usually the first 12 days of the calendar month for ease.

The estrogen dose should be strong enough to relieve hot flashes and maintain bone strength. For most women this corresponds to a daily dose of Premarin equal to 0.625 milligrams, oral estradiol dose of 1 milligram, or transdermal dose of 0.05 milligrams. If hot flashes are not relieved, the dose can be increased in increments until symptoms resolve.

The progestagen dose should be sufficient to counteract potential estrogen hyperstimulation in the uterus. (If you've had a hysterectomy, progestagen is not needed—don't take it.) Continuous regimens could include 2.5 milligrams of medroxyprogesterone each day or the equivalent micro-nized progesterone dose of 100 milligrams daily. CombiPatch, which is a continuous method in a transdermal system, provides 0.05 milligrams of estradiol and 0.14 milligrams of norethindrone acetate.

Your need for local (vaginal) vs. systemic therapy: If you have excellent bone density, no cardiac risk factors, no family history of breast cancer, and no major hot flash symptoms, you may want to only treat the symptom of vaginal atrophy. As long as you use a minimal amount of estrogen (Estring, Premarin cream 0.625 milligrams per week, or estradiol cream 0.5 milligrams per week) you will not develop systemic effects and will not need to take a progestagen. Conversely, you will not get any benefit to the heart or bones as you would from systemic therapy.

Desire for natural or traditional therapy: Once you've read this chapter, talked to your doctor, discussed the issues with your friends, and "surfed the net" you may find that one of these approaches appeals to you more than the other. While most of our research and current knowledge pertains to traditional therapy, natural medicines are gaining popularity as studies fail to show major disadvantages. Keep in mind that most of the information we are getting from studies is ongoing with new information appearing in medical journals on a regular basis. The next five years are sure to offer an explosion of information.

Ease of use: Sometimes easy is just better. Some regimens are more involved than others, demanding intricate schedules or difficult administration. Sometimes side effects such as stomach upset from an oral medication, skin irritation from a transdermal application, or vaginal discharge from creams or the ring may be more trouble than they are worth.

Cost: As is often the case, sometimes money is the bottom line. You may be financially limited to medications that your health insurance will accept. If this is not a factor, you will find a large difference in cost for various therapies. Generic medications are almost always less expensive than brand name products.

Finally, don't be discouraged if you don't feel satisfied with the first regimen you try. Sometimes it is a matter of trial and error, which is acceptable as long as you take hormones in doses adequate to do the job they're meant to do and don't leave yourself vulnerable to over-stimulation of the uterus. You can combine transdermal estrogens and oral progestagens or you may need to adjust your dosing schedule if you have spotting or bleeding, but always check with your doctor first before making a change. The bottom line is that you should feel confident and comfortable with the medicine you are taking.

The following is a sampling of popular regimens for conventional HRT:

- Premarin 0.625 milligrams (or estradiol 0.5 milligrams) on days 1 to 25 of the calendar month with the addition of medroxyprogesterone 10 milligrams on days 16 to 25; no medication is taken for the remainder of the month, which is when bleeding will occur.

- Premarin 0.625 milligrams (or estradiol 0.5 milligrams) each day of the month with the addition of medroxyprogesterone on days 1 to 12 of the calendar month. Expect bleeding shortly after day 12.

- PremPro 0.625/2.5 or PremPro 0.625/5: These are combined regimens containing 0.625 milligrams of Premarin with either 2.5 or 5 milligrams of medroxyprogesterone in the *same* pill. There should be no bleeding with this continuous method.

- PremPhase 0.625/5: This is a prepackaged cyclic regimen in which the first 14 days consists only of Premarin 0.625 milligrams and the last 14 days contains the same Premarin dose plus medroxyprogesterone 5 milligrams. Expect bleeding after the last combined hormone pill on day 28.

- Transdermal estradiol patch delivering 0.05 milligrams of estradiol each day with the addition of medroxyprogesterone either continuously (dose of 2.5 milligrams) or cyclically (dose of 10 milligrams for 10 to 14 days each

Watch Out!
If you forget to take a dose of medication or travel through several times zones, thus throwing your body off its normal rhythm, you may start to bleed. This is not alarming as long as the bleeding is clearly related to a missed pill or change in time zones. In these cases your body is smarter than you are. Prolonged unanticipated bleeding should always be discussed with your physician.

month). Patches are applied twice weekly, the exceptions being Climara and FemPatch, which are applied once per week.

■ Tri-Est 1.25 milligram capsule (contains estriol 1.0 milligram, estradiol 0.125 milligrams, and estrone 0.125 milligrams) taken daily with natural progesterone capsule 100 milligrams also taken daily. Expect no bleeding.

■ Estratest HS can substitute for an estrogen in any of the above regimens (except PremPro or PremPhase). Add a progestin as above.

■ CombiPatch transdermal patch is applied twice weekly and should not cause bleeding. It supplies estradiol 0.05 milligrams and norethindrone acetate 0.14 milligrams each day.

This is not an exhaustive list but is meant to show some of the common combinations used in clinical practice. There is no doubt that the list of available medications will grow with time.

HRT, medications, and existing ailments

Conditions that you already have, such as high blood pressure or liver disease, can interact negatively with your HRT regimen. For some conditions, however, prescribing a certain type of estrogen or progestin (or a certain method of taking it) may actually *help*.

It's important to talk with your physician about any personal or family history of disease so that you can settle on the best plan for your health. Also show your doctor a list of the medications that you take regularly because a wide range of medications can affect hormone-replacement therapy (or be affected by it).

Estrogen and . . .

Check package inserts, and discuss with your physician how taking certain medications can affect the estrogen part of your HRT regimen. Prescription drugs that may alter the way that your body uses estrogen include the following:

- Drugs that potentially damage the liver; Acetaminophen (such as Tylenol, when taken in high dosages), Tegretol, Chloroquine, Depakote

- Acetaminophen (such as Tylenol), in high dosages and for extended use

- Amiodarone (such as Cordarone)

- Anabolic steroids (nandrolone, such as Anabolin; oxandrolone, such as Anavar; oxymetholone, such as Anadrol; and stanozolol, such as Winstrol)

- Androgens

- Anti-infectives

- Antithyroid agents, which are used to treat hyperthyroidism

- Carbamazepine (such as Tegretol)

- Carmustine (such as BiCNU)

- Chloroquine (such as Aralen)

- Cyclosporine (such as Sandimmune) because estrogens may retard cyclosporine's removal from the body, resulting in kidney or liver problems

- Dantrolene (such as Dantrium)

- Daunorubicin (such as Cerubidine)

- Disulfiram (such as Antabuse)

- Divalproex (such as Depakote)

- Etretinate (such as Tegison)

- Gold salts, which are used to treat arthritis

- Hydroxychloroquine (such as Plaquenil)

- Isoniazid

- Mercaptopurine (such as Purinethol)

- Methotrexate (such as Mexate)

- Methyldopa (such as Aldomet)

- Naltrexone (such as Trexan), for long-term, high-dose use

- Oral contraceptives containing estrogen (most)

- Phenothiazines (acetophenazine, such as Tindal; chlorpromazine, such as Thorazine; fluphenazine, such as Prolixin; mesoridazine, such as Serentil; perphenazine, such as Trilafon; prochlorperazine, such as Compazine; promazine, such as Sparine; promethazine, such as Phenergan; thioridazine, such as Mellaril; trifluoperazine, such as Stelazine; triflupromazine, such as Vesprin; and trime-prazine, such as Temaril)

- Phenytoin (such as Dilantin)

- Plicamycin (such as Mithracin)

- Protease inhibitors such as ritonavir (such as Norvir, which may decrease the estrogen effect)

- Valproic acid (such as Depakene), which may increase the chance of liver problems in combined use with estrogens

Before you select an HRT regimen, you should let your doctor know whether you have any of the following health conditions:

- Problems with blood clotting

- Problems with oral contraceptives or other forms of hormone administration

Watch Out!
Always check with your physician first if you want to make changes in your regimen and/or if you experience notable side effects.

- Breast, bone, or uterine cancer
- Uterine fibroids
- Changes in uterine bleeding patterns without known cause
- Endometriosis
- High cholesterol
- High triglycerides
- Gallbladder disease or gallstones
- Liver disease
- Pancreatitis

Watch Out!
You should *not* use estrogen if you are pregnant. Estrogen therapy has been associated with increased risk of birth defects in the reproductive organs of a fetus, as well as with vaginal and cervical disease in the female later in life.

Administering estrogen can make diagnosing uterine-bleeding problems difficult, so your doctor may want to delay estrogen therapy until more is known about any odd bleeding patterns that you experience. Estrogens can potentially worsen certain cancers, such as breast or endometrial cancer. Estrogens can also exacerbate certain inflammatory conditions, liver disease, asthma, migraine headaches, fibroid tumors of the uterus, and gallstones. They may worsen blood-triglyceride profiles and may occasionally exacerbate high blood pressure in some women.

Progestins and progesterone
The following drugs can interfere with the way that your body uses progestins:

- Aminoglutethimide (Cytadren)
- Carbamazepine (Tegretol)
- Phenobarbital
- Phenytoin (Dilantin)
- Rifabutin (Mycobutin)
- Rifampin (Rifadin, Rimactane)

If you have a history of any of the following conditions, be sure to discuss with your physician how progestin (or progesterone) use might affect them:

- Asthma

- Epilepsy

- Heart or circulation difficulties

- Severe kidney disease

- Migraine headaches

- Undiagnosed bleeding problems (because the use of progestins can make some bleeding conditions more difficult to diagnose)

- Breast disease (including lumps or cysts)

- Depression

- Diabetes (because progestins may cause a slight increase in blood sugar, requiring adjustment of your diabetes medication)

- High cholesterol (which progestins may make cause or worsen)

- Liver disease (which can be worsened by certain progestin effects)

- Osteoporosis or conditions increasing chances of osteoporosis (because certain progestin doses may cause temporary bone thinning)

Should you become pregnant while taking progestins, progesterone, or any form of HRT, inform your prescribing doctor immediately. Although progesterone is often called "the pregnancy hormone" because your body makes so much of it when you're pregnant, there have been reports that some progestins may cause birth defects, including low birth weight and inappropriate masculinizing or feminizing of fetal genitalia.

Watch Out!
Progestins can exacerbate migraine headaches by encouraging fluid buildup.

Always try to stay in touch with your body, note any adverse effects (even if they seem to be unconnected to HRT), and tell your doctor about any problems. HRT affects a wide range of tissues and functions in the female body in both negative and positive ways. Remember that if your HRT regimen doesn't fit quite right, the dosage, administration method, or type of hormone can be tweaked to give you a comfortable fit.

Just the facts

- Different types of hormones and ways of taking them can create different results and side effects.

- Progestins may behave differently in the body than natural progesterone.

- Non-oral forms of hormone administration tend to provide more physiologic dosages—orally administered hormones require higher dosages due to the body's metabolization.

- Oral hormones require higher dosages since they must first be absorbed by the stomach and are not absorbed directly into the bloodstream. Non-oral forms, once absorbed are picked up by the blood stream, require lower doses, and tend to mimic the body's natural hormones.

- In the United States, most women who undergo estrogen replacement take Premarin.

GET THE SCOOP ON...
Bone protection ▪ Designer estrogens and
antihormones ▪ Estrogenlike treatments
and the risk of breast cancer ▪ What's
new in pharmaceuticals

New Drugs and Designer Hormones

Chapter 9

Conventional medicine offers more than just hormone-replacement therapy to assist a woman through difficult menopause and to help prevent conditions for which postmenopausal women are at risk. In fact, what you might call *antihormones* are now part of the pharmaceutical cornucopia, as are so-called *designer hormones*— hormonelike pharmaceuticals that target specific actions in the body.

When would a woman want to consider these substances instead of regular HRT? When she needs potentially greater protection than conventional hormone-replacement therapy offers and when she needs to diminish certain HRT risks. If she's at particularly high risk of developing osteoporosis or breast cancer, for example, specific hormone-related treatment options can greatly reduce her risk.

Also, taking designer estrogens as hormone-replacement therapy may prevent the need for an additional progestin prescription because designer estrogens aren't always associated with the increased cancer risks that progestins are used to counter. (Also remember that some women don't tolerate progestin therapy well.) These facts are especially important because four of every five women who use regular HRT discontinue taking hormones within two years, largely because of side effects such as bleeding, as well as concern about increased risk of certain cancers.

This chapter introduces the main designer hormones and antihormones, tells you what they're used for, describes how they work, and discusses who should and shouldn't consider taking them.

Designer estrogens to prevent osteoporosis

Unofficially... Recent research shows that half the usual dose of estrogen may be enough to keep osteoporosis away from post-menopausal women. The reduced dose may also mean lower breast-cancer risk while still maintaining protection from heart disease.

As you see in Chapter 8, different types of estrogens (or, for that matter, progestins or progesterone) have slightly different effects in the body, and physicians prescribing HRT find that their patients may even feel better on one type instead of another. In the female body, the hormones known as estrogens are really a group of hormones lumped under the heading "estrogens." You may as well think of estrogens as being a variety of flavors and estrogen receptors being sensitive taste buds.

Researchers have gone far beyond plain-vanilla estrogen. Among the more exotic estrogen flavors today is raloxifene hydrochloride (best known by the trade name EVISTA), which the U.S. Food and Drug Administration approved in 1997. This estrogen is specifically designed to prevent osteoporosis and is used only by postmenopausal women who are not using other estrogens.

Raloxifene and how it works

As discussed in Chapter 4 there are estrogen receptors in practically all of the body's cells. Estrogen has a specific shape that fits perfectly into these receptors. In this way, estrogen acts like a master key and the receptors act like the many locks that it can open. If the shape of a designer estrogen compound is similar enough to the body's natural estrogen, it can bind to an estrogen receptor. These designer estrogens will do one of two things when they bind to a receptor. They either stimulate the receptor as estrogen does, literally opening the door to estrogen activity, or they bind to the receptor without provoking the cascade of estrogen reactions.

In this last case, the modified estrogen binds to the receptor yet does not result in estrogen activity. In addition it *prevents* natural estrogen from attaching to the receptor, thus blocking its ability to stimulate the receptor. This concept of selective activity is very important in understanding this group of estrogens. As a group, these compounds are called selective estrogen receptor modulators or SERMs. With the advent of raloxifene these compounds have been established as a group unto themselves, but as we'll see later in this chapter SERMs have been in existence for several decades.

The selective effect of raloxifene and other SERMs is due to the existence of different types of estrogen receptors. These receptors were only discovered several years ago and future research may very well reveal several more. The existing receptors are called alpha receptors and beta receptors. Alpha receptors are located in the reproductive organs such as the breast, uterus, and vagina.

Beta receptors are located in bone and blood vessels. Estrogen stimulates both types of receptors whereas raloxifene seems to activate only the beta receptors.

Like other estrogens, raloxifene stops postmenopausal bone loss by binding to hormone receptors in bone that prevent its resorption (remodeling of bone with a loss of bone mass), albeit to a lesser extent than estrogen. By blocking resorption into the system, the levels of circulating calcium in the body are slightly boosted, and bone density improves. While raloxifene has been found to halt progression of bone loss, it hasn't yet been conclusively found to *reverse* existing osteoporosis.

Unlike typical estrogens, raloxifene doesn't stimulate receptors in the breast or uterus. Therefore, it is not believed to increase the risk of cancer in those tissues. (Clinical studies of EVISTA, conducted for two-and-a-half years, found that the risk for breast or endometrial cancer did not increase.)

During a two-year clinical trial funded by Eli Lilly, the manufacturers of EVISTA, to investigate the effects of the medicine on osteoporosis, an interesting finding was made. The group of 7,700 women using raloxifene had 70 percent fewer new breast cancers than similarly matched women in the control group who took only a placebo. While exciting, this information has to be interpreted with caution. It is believed that it takes breast cancers at least five years from the time of their inception to the point of their detection. If this is true, it is unclear if raloxifene is merely slowing growth of existing tumors or actually preventing them from occurring. Perhaps it will have no impact at all on breast cancer incidence, but will merely increase the time interval from tumor origin to the time when it is detected.

Perhaps the rate of breast cancer will even increase after several years of raloxifene use. While this is unlikely, the answer to this and the preceding questions is unknown at this time. In any event, it is an area of intense interest that is being further investigated.

Raloxifene has similar but not equal effects as compared to estrogen on bone mineral density and cholesterol. These effects were reported in *The New England Journal of Medicine* in December of 1997. Over a two-year period of time, average bone mineral density in the total body was increased by 2 percent. Estrogen has been shown to increase bone mineral density by 4 to 5 percent. Numerous studies have shown beneficial cholesterol changes with raloxifene albeit not as favorable as those of estrogen. Raloxifene decreases LDL, the bad cholesterol and decreases total cholesterol levels; but it does not decrease HDL, the good cholesterol.

Since raloxifene does not stimulate breast receptors, users do not experience the typical HRT-related annoyance of breast tenderness. Similarly, raloxifene does not stimulate receptors in the uterus, thus eliminating another major HRT annoyance: bleeding. This eliminates the need to take a progestin as well. Women taking raloxifene only need to take one pill each and every day—a "no brainer." Preliminary studies show no increase in the risk of endometrial cancer.

Lack of receptor stimulation in other areas may be a detriment to raloxifene use for some women. Since it does not affect the vagina, raloxifene may not be suitable for those women with severe vaginal dryness and urogenital atrophy. Raloxifene does not relieve hot flashes, and it does not appear to improve skin texture, as does estrogen.

Watch Out! The FDA has issued a notice regarding the prescribing of EVISTA (raloxifene HC1, the product described in this chapter), after receiving numerous reports noting confusion between it and an unrelated pharmaceutical called E-Vista (a generic form of hydroxyzine HC1), which was formerly manufactured by Seatrace Pharmaceuticals, Inc. and which is still listed in some prescription drug guides. Make sure the prescription you get and fill is correct!

The beneficial characteristics of raloxifene include the following:

- It has been found to have a protective effect on bone density.

- It lowers blood levels of total and LDL (bad) cholesterol but doesn't raise triglycerides or HDL (good) cholesterol.

- It doesn't stimulate breast or uterine tissue, as other estrogens do.

Studies of bone-mineral density compared the daily use of 60 milligrams of EVISTA with the use of a calcium-supplemented placebo by women who had hysterectomies. After two years, the EVISTA group was found to have average bone density up to 2 percent higher than that of the control group.

The drawbacks

The decision to use raloxifene instead of or in conjunction with hormone-replacement therapy is a matter for you and your doctor to discuss. Table 9.1 shows who should and who should not consider taking it.

Note! ➜
If you're seriously considering using raloxifene, read about it at Eli Lilly & Co.'s Web site about EVISTA (www.evista. com), or ask your pharmacist or physician for a full package insert.

TABLE 9.1: RALOXIFENE USE

Indicated [Candidate for use]	Contraindicated [Not candidate for use]
If you want to prevent osteoporosis	If you have a history of blood clots
If you are postmenopausal	If you have liver disease
If you are at increased risk of cardiovascular disease	If you suffer from extended immobility
If you are at increased risk of breast cancer	If you are pregnant
	If you are already taking estrogen-replacement therapy

Most of the conditions that are contraindications for raloxifene use are identical to those for estrogen use. Women who are pregnant should not take it, for example, because raloxifene can harm a fetus. (Because the drug is prescribed for postmenopausal women, however, this situation shouldn't be a problem.) Women who have blood clots or even a family history of blood clots shouldn't take raloxifene, either. When estrogens and SERMs are taken orally, they are metabolized (broken down) by the liver. This stimulates the liver to manufacture extra clotting factors which then increases the likelihood of blood clots forming in veins. Neither should the drug be taken by women who will be immobile for a long time (such as during an illness that requires prolonged bed rest) because of increased risk of clotting. Women who have liver disease are also not candidates for these hormones because a well functioning liver is needed to safely process these medicines.

If any of these conditions affects you, discuss it with your doctor before you decide on raloxifene. Also discuss your other medical conditions, such as congestive heart failure or active cancer.

If you're taking raloxifene, be sure to tell your doctor if you experience any of the following:

- Swelling of hands, feet, or legs
- Abnormal vaginal bleeding
- Breast pain or enlargement
- Pregnancy

Despite raloxifene's benefits for some women, the most widely prescribed traditional estrogen, Premarin, has been found to be significantly better at improving bone-mineral density. Wyeth-Ayerst,

Moneysaver
Another drawback to raloxifene is cost. A daily dose of 60 milligrams can cost about $70 per month. Comparable prescriptions of conventional estrogen replacements cost about 40 percent less.

Watch Out!
If you're taking blood thinners (such as warfarin or other coumarin preparations), check with your doctor before taking raloxifene because your medication may need to be adjusted.

the maker of Premarin, reports that during a two-year study, mineral density of the hip bones increased three times more in patients who were taking Premarin than in those who were given raloxifene.

You can't take raloxifene to alleviate the common symptoms of menopause; it works only on bone and doesn't help hot flashes. Unfortunately, women who were taking EVISTA had a higher incidence of hot flashes than those who were taking a placebo—25 percent versus 18 percent. Most of the time, this situation occurred early in treatment rather than after the first six months. Leg cramps were also more frequent in EVISTA takers, with 6 percent of women in that group reporting cramping versus 2 percent in the placebo group.

Currently, raloxifene has received FDA approval only for use in preventing osteoporosis in post-menopausal women. The drug is, like other SERMs, being studied for other disease-preventative uses, however. The effectiveness of raloxifene in reducing breast cancer risk has not been *established,* but very preliminary data suggests that raloxifene *may* have the potential to significantly reduce breast-cancer risk.

1998 interim results of the ongoing multicenter MORE (Multiple Outcomes of Raloxifene Evaluation) study showed more than a 50 percent reduction in the incidence of breast cancer among women enrolled in ongoing osteoporosis studies and taking raloxifene, and other data suggests the preventative benefit could potentially exceed 70 percent. Further studies are being conducted to explore the possibility.

A boon for breast cancer prevention

Another widely discussed SERM is tamoxifen (trade name Nolvadex, manufactured by Zeneca). Tamoxifen is a pill that interferes with the activity of estrogen and therefore might be called an *antiestrogen*. The drug has been used for more than two decades in the treatment of advanced breast cancer and has been shown to be beneficial as a treatment during early stages of the disease.

Recently, tamoxifen has been studied as a preventative treatment for women who are at high risk of developing breast cancer. In one study subjects who took it were found to have less than half the breast-cancer incidence of those who didn't—a remarkable risk reduction.

However there is some conflicting data. Researchers in Italy and England report in their studies tamoxifen did not appear to prevent breast cancer. Additional studies of the drug's breast cancer preventative benefits are being conducted.

The FDA is convinced enough of tamoxifen's beneficial use that it is approved for the reduction in the incidence of breast cancer in women at high risk for developing the disease, among its other indications.

Although tamoxifen is helping save the lives of breast-cancer patients, it isn't a panacea. Tamoxifen, in fact, carries its own serious risks. A breast-cancer prevention trial sponsored by the National Cancer Institute studied more than 13,000 women who used the drug as a preventative; the women who took tamoxifen had a higher risk of uterine cancer and pulmonary embolus (blood clots in the lungs).

Bright Idea
You can take a short online quiz to determine your own risk of different reproductive cancers. To find the interactive quiz, visit the Women's Cancer Network Web site (www.wcn.org/risk/).

Despite the drug's dramatic protective effects, caution is advised in prescribing it. In 1994 the FDA issued a stronger warning on tamoxifen following new studies linking it to a rate of uterine cancer two to three times higher than the risk for women without breast cancer in the general population.

You can expect to hear more about tamoxifen and its potential use, particularly for women at high risk of developing breast cancer but low risk of developing uterine cancer and blood clots.

Taking tamoxifen

This book has already discussed the links between high estrogen levels and potential breast cancer. How does it work and why do SERMs hold promise?

Estrogen has a proliferative effect on some cells, including certain breast-cancer cells. The hormone binds to the cells and prompts them to grow and increase in number. In susceptible persons this increased growth effect may be the necessary stimulus for development and proliferation of breast cancer.

Breast cancers are diverse. Some tumors have a high affinity for estrogen and are termed "estrogen receptor positive." Others are "estrogen receptor negative" and do not appear to grow as a result of increased estrogen. To muddy the waters even further, some breast cancers are progesterone receptor positive and some are progesterone receptor negative.

With the advent of SERMs, with their anti-estrogen properties, as well as some new anti-progesterone drugs that will be discussed later in this chapter, this information takes on a whole new dimension to the postmenopausal woman.

Tamoxifen, like raloxifene, is a selective estrogen receptor modulator (SERM). It prevents estrogen from binding to the cells and thereby thwarts the hormone's capability to stimulate cancer growth. Tamoxifen has been used as an anti-estrogen treatment for breast cancer for more than twenty years. It was originally used for breast cancer treatment in those women with positive estrogen receptors and spread of the tumor to the lymph nodes in the armpit. Over time it became obvious that women without spread to the lymph nodes would also benefit from its use.

In April of 1998 the National Cancer Institute stopped a 5-year study on the effects of tamoxifen as a *preventive medication* for breast cancer one year early because they felt it was unethical to withhold this medicine from the placebo group. The study compared women at high risk of developing breast cancer, as determined by risk factor analysis, and divided them into two groups: One group received a placebo (no medicine), and the other group received tamoxifen. They found the tamoxifen group had a 44 percent reduced risk of invasive breast cancer as compared to the placebo group. The reduced risk was seen only in estrogen-positive breast tumors. The results of this study led the Food and Drug Administration (FDA) to expand tamoxifen's approved use to include *reduction of the incidence of breast cancer.* This is the first time the FDA has approved a drug to reduce the incidence of a cancer!

Women who fit into the category of high risk for this study included the following:

- Age greater than or equal to 60 years.

- Age greater than or equal to 35 years with previous lobular caricinoma in situ (a form of early, noninvasive breast cancer).

Bright Idea
You can contact a toll free number 1-800-34-LIFE-4 supported by Zeneca, the makers of Nolvadex, to obtain free information on Nolvadex, breast cancer, and prevention of the disease in healthy women. In addition to printed material a video is also available.

- Age greater than or equal to 35 years with a combination of the following risk factors:

  Number of first-degree relatives with breast cancer

  History and number of breast biopsies

  History of atypical hyperplasia (a forerunner of breast cancer)

  Early age at first period

  Late age at first birth or no children at all

But tamoxifen isn't a total anti-estrogen. In fact, elsewhere in the body, it behaves like a weak estrogen. As a result, it may help prevent osteoporosis and heart disease, as well as confer other benefits of estrogen therapy.

Using a weak estrogen to ameliorate the unwanted effects of stronger estrogens is also partly why plant estrogens (known as *phytoestrogens*) are of such interest. Many of these plant estrogens exert weaker hormonal activity than the main human estrogen, estradiol. The same may be said of estriol, a weaker human estrogen that is popularly prescribed in Europe (and prescribed in the United States for women seeking HRT who are at higher-than-normal risk of breast cancer).

Tough trade-offs

It's a tough trade-off if tamoxifen can help breast cancer but make other conditions just as bad or potentially worse. Although 45 percent of women studied were found to have reduced incidence of breast cancer when they took tamoxifen, two patients died from blood clots in their lungs. As mentioned earlier in this chapter, the risk of endometrial cancer also increases in women who take tamoxifen (but less often (1 percent) if using only 20 milligrams daily).

As is the case with most medications, tamoxifen has potential risks and benefits. The medicine has clearly been shown to be beneficial in reducing the incidence of breast cancer progression and seems to decrease the development of breast cancer in women at high risk for this cancer.

A small percentage of women who take this drug will develop endometrial cancer. This form of cancer is generally very treatable and is usually detected in its early stage if warning signs are heeded. Any woman taking tamoxifen who has bleeding should be evaluated with an endometrial biopsy. This is an office procedure during which a thin, flexible plastic device is threaded past the cervix (opening of the uterus) and into the uterine cavity. Samples of the uterine lining (endometrium) are then quickly suctioned up so that they can be sent to the pathology lab for analysis. In this way abnormalities can be detected and evaluated. In addition to endometrial cancer, tamoxifen use is associated with two benign conditions, endometrial polyps and adenomatous hyperplasia (an overgrowth phenomenon).

Tamoxifen has a few side effects. It may actually induce menopause in perimenopausal women, and it can cause symptoms such as hot flashes, irregular menstruation, vaginal dryness, weight gain, mood fluctuations, or depression. If you take tamoxifen, you also may be at slightly greater risk of developing cataracts (or your existing cataracts may worsen).

If you take tamoxifen, you should do the following things:

■ Have regular gynecological exams.

■ Have an opthalmological exam every two years.

Tamoxifen isn't necessarily a lifelong commitment, although its effects may last many years after
you stop taking it. Benefits have occurred in women
even 15 years after they started using the drug and
10 years after they stopped. The exact length of time
for which tamoxifen should be taken when used as
treatment for breast cancer is a matter of individual
judgment, although studies have focused on a
five-year period of taking the drug. Appropriate
guidelines for *preventive* use in women without
breast cancer using this SERM as a form of HRT are
evolving as more research is done.

Tamoxifen isn't the only drug that can be called
an anti-estrogen (although as mentioned earlier in
this chapter, it has selective estrogenic effects, too).
Anastrozole (trade name Arimidex by Zeneca) was
approved in 1996 for the treatment of postmenopausal breast cancer that has progressed following therapy with tamoxifen. The drug is not a
steroid, but an aromatase inhibitor that cuts down
the *production* of estrogen.

Summing up SERMs

New pharmaceuticals that target women's health
issues are being developed, and existing medicines
are being tested for new applications.

Raloxifene, for example, is being evaluated
for possible use in preventing breast cancer and
cardiovascular disease. Other SERMs—such as
droloxifene, levomeloxifene, and idoxifene—are
being tested as well for potential use in preventing
osteoporosis and breast cancer.

As researchers probe deeper into the workings
of the body's hormonal systems, they learned more
about how estrogen works in the body. Rather than
estrogen's fitting into estrogen receptors like a

simple key into a lock, for example, investigators now think that synthetic hormones can change the estrogen receptor's shape and influence gene expression, interacting with different bits of DNA, depending on their configuration.

SERMs like tamoxifen (the first widely used one) and raloxifene have been described as being *intentionally defective* estrogen keys. These SERMs can fit into a lock (the estrogen receptor) but can't always perform all the duties of regular estrogens, so they act selectively.

Tamoxifen, for example, is a key that fits the estrogen-receptor locks in breast tissue, thereby blocking the keyholes from binding with circulating estrogen. But this SERM's happy defect is its failure to stimulate the growth of breast tissue as normal estrogen would, so it has protective effects against breast cancer. Existing cancer of the breast is deprived of the estrogen upon which it normally relies, and new cancer is not prompted.

Tamoxifen's selective action in the body means that it can accomplish some of the good things normally done by estrogen: reducing cholesterol, for example, and warding off osteoporosis. Less fortunately, it does *not* prevent cell growth in uterine tissue. There, in effect, it mimics the behavior of estrogen, and in fact women who take tamoxifen run a somewhat increased chance of developing endometrial cancer over women without the medicine.

New SERMs with even more selectivity are being developed in the hope of getting the lock-and-key combination just right, producing the intended effects without *unwanted* estrogenic effects. The SERM raloxifene, which is currently approved solely for osteoporosis prevention but is being evaluated

Bright Idea
If you are interested in taking part in clinical trials for new cancer treatments, you can find out more at the National Cancer Institute's Web site (http://cancertrials.nci.nih.gov/) or via the organization's Cancer Information Service, at 1-800-4-CANCER.

for other uses, prevents estrogen from binding to estrogen receptors in both breast and uterine tissue, so it is not expected to increase the risk of cancer in those areas. Longer duration studies with larger numbers of subjects are needed to reach this conclusion.

You can easily see why SERMs are a fascinating area of study and why they can potentially help many women. Yet the use of these drugs in the population at large is still new, and researchers want to learn about the long-term effects of taking them.

SERMs being studied for further uses include Eli Lilly & Co.'s EVISTA (raloxifene), droloxifene (Pfizer; for breast cancer), CP-336,156 (also by Pfizer), and others that are being worked on by Wyeth-Ayerst. A Swedish biotech company called KaroBio is studying what molecules may trigger a newly discovered type of estrogen receptor called the beta receptor (described earlier in this chapter).

More interesting things are being learned about estrogen's activity in the body—such as the fact that it can take any of three pathways in the body. This discovery affirms estrogen's widespread action in different organ systems. Future SERMs may target not only specific receptors, but also just a single estrogen pathway, creating even more precise effects.

The challenge of using SERMs—and perhaps the major point to evaluate if you're considering taking them—is getting the estrogen effects that you want, *not* the ones that you don't. Also, traditional hormone-replacement therapy has the benefit of longer-term testing related to menopause issues.

Antiprogestins and postmenopausal health

Unofficially...
Every 64 minutes, on average, a woman in the United States is diagnosed with cancer of the reproductive organs.

After all this talk about so-called antiestrogens, you may be interested to know *antiprogestins* are also being studied. Endocrinological researchers are hailing antiprogestins as being among the most significant recent scientific developments in their field. Although several hundred such compounds have been made in the laboratory, only a few have been tested in animals or humans, and you may know the name of only one (RU-486 (mifepristone), often termed the *French abortion pill*). According to a 1995 review of antiprogestins by researchers with the World Health Organization in Switzerland, at that time, only these three antiprogestins had been tested in humans:

- Mifepristone (RU-486)

- Lilopristone (ZK 98.734)

- Onapristone (ZK 98.299)

- Uterine fibroids

The following list shows some of the myriad uses for antiprogestins beyond abortion agents.

- Menses induction (when used
  with a prostaglandin, in fertility regulation)

- Contraception (by ovulation inhibition)

- Meningiomas (brain tumors)

- Endometriosis

- Uterine fibroids

- Labor induction in delivery

- Breast cancer

- Ovarian cancer

How may antiprogestins work, say, in the case of breast cancer? Some breast cancers depend on the actions of progesterone, and antiprogestin research may lead to a treatment for many of those tumors. By binding to and blocking progesterone receptors, antiprogestins may be able to slow the cancer's growth rate or possibly reduce tumors.

Although they are pleased by the development of antiprogestin study, researchers who are reviewing the possible future uses of antiprogestins say that for scientific and practical reasons, a new generation of more-specific antihormones is desirable. Early generation drugs antiprogestins acted against the glucocortoid hormones as well. Preferably, molecules will be developed that have either antiprogestational or antiglucocorticoid capabilities—not both. This would allow for more specific actions of the compounds with fewer side effects. There is no doubt that a selective antiprogestin would be useful in treating menopausal conditions or hormone dependent breast tumors in menopausal women.

Beyond designer sex hormones

Protecting women's bones is a potentially huge pharmaceutical market, and drug researchers and manufacturers are by no means limiting their work to developing designer hormones.

Nonhormonal therapies offer much to women who can't or won't undergo HRT or use designer estrogens, as well as to those who want to use conventional HRT but prefer some extra protection.

Bone benefits

Another new osteoporosis product is the antiresorptive (prevents breakdown of bone) medication alendronate (trade name Fosamax, developed by Merck & Co.). Alendronate, which is specifically designed for use by postmenopausal women, is the first nonhormonal therapy for osteoporosis. By inhibiting the breakdown of skeletal bone, alendronate can not only cut the loss of bone, but also increase bone mass.

The drug doesn't appear to increase breast-cancer risk because it acts only on bone. A study of more than 1,600 women in the United States, Great Britain, and Denmark found that estrogen and alendronate increased spinal density by 3 percent to 4 percent annually.

Bisphosphonates are not a new category of drug; Etidronate and Pamidronate have been used for years for a variety of disorders related to calcium and bone. Those drugs are not appropriate for long-term use in treating osteoporosis, however, due to some of their other effects. Alendronate is a safer drug in the same category and is appropriate for longer-term use.

Some people who have taken alendronate reported gastrointestinal distress, ranging from abdominal pain and nausea to diarrhea or constipation, gas, and even ulcers. Headaches and musculoskeletal pain have also been reported. To allow the drug's absorption and prevent distress, you should not lie down for half an hour after taking it

A study in the *New England Journal of Medicine* in February 1998 investigated whether or not lower doses of alendronate could be effective and better tolerated. They found a dose of 5 milligrams per day was well tolerated with a large reduction in side effects and was as effective as HRT in maintaining bone density. Thus, the 5 milligram dose is acceptable for women who have osteopenia (bone thinning not severe enough to be labeled osteoporosis) or want to maintain their current level without the

Watch Out!
One peculiarity of alendronate is how it should be taken: on an empty stomach with water about half an hour before a meal. Even coffee or certain vitamin/mineral supplements taken with it can dramatically reduce its absorption and effectiveness.

use of HRT. For women with severe loss as is seen with osteoporosis, the larger 10 milligram dose gives superior results.

Four multiple-year studies of alendronate in postmenopausal women who had osteoporosis found that 10 milligrams a day can increase the density of bone and cut the rate of fractures in older women. Use of the drug has even correlated with a decrease in the height loss that occurs with aging. (The studies included a daily 500-milligram calcium supplement, however.)

Gone fishing?

Miacalcin nasal spray (calcitonin-salmon), developed by Sandoz Pharmaceuticals, is an osteoporosis treatment for women at least five years past menopause who have low bone-mass density and can't take estrogens. The *salmon* in *calcitonin-salmon* refers to the fish.

Calcitonin is actually a hormone, not exclusive to the human set, that is secreted by the thyroid gland. But the sturdy salmon's version of calcitonin, it seems, works in humans at almost 30 times the potency of our own calcitonin.

A main effect of the spray is the inhibition of osteoclasts: cells that transport calcium out of the bone. By preventing bone loss, calcitonin allows stronger, more solid bone to form.

The nasal spray is taken along with a daily dose of 1,000 milligrams of elemental calcium and 400 IU of vitamin D. See Chapter 10 for explanation of these terms.

In the pipeline

Pharmaceutical researchers are continuing to work on appropriate osteoporosis preventatives and treatments. New generations of SERMs look promising

Unofficially...
Calcitonin is found in a specific gland of the fish in question. You can't obtain it from a salmon fillet!

in that regard. Even parathyroid hormone is being looked at as a potential osteoporosis treatment.

New drugs are being developed to treat other problems that may affect postmenopausal women. Urinary incontinence, for example, is believed to affect 15 percent to 35 percent of people over 60 and to affect twice as many women as men. The likelihood of incontinence increases greatly in the homebound elderly.

Although existing drugs are used to treat the condition, two new ones may be promising. Tolterodine tartrate (Detrol), developed by Pharmacia & Upjohn, was approved by the FDA in 1998 for treatment of patients with an overactive bladder with symptoms of urinary frequency, urgency, or urge incontinence. Duloxetine, which is being developed by Eli Lilly & Co., is undergoing evaluation for use against urinary incontinence.

Tolterodine tartrate works primarily on receptors in the bladder to reduce urination urges. Duloxetine works similarly to popular antidepressants; it is reported to inhibit reuptake of serotonin and norepinephrine. In its actions on the central nervous system, duloxetine stimulates sphincter motor neurons thereby decreasing involuntary urine loss.

If you see the potential benefits of a new therapy for serious conditions and are willing to forge into new territory, you may have an option beyond visiting your physician. By enrolling in a clinical human trial to test treatments in development, you may not only gain access to a drug that is not yet on the market for the general public, but also may gain free medical care and testing (in addition to the drug). Although the decision to participate in a human trial is certainly not one to be taken lightly, drugs

Watch Out!
If you're interested in trying a new pharmaceutical, be sure to discuss it thoroughly with your physician. Although new generations of drugs offer great promise, there hasn't been time to see what happens with truly long-term use. Established therapies can be considered to be more tried and true.

that reach the evaluation stage in humans have already undergone substantial testing in animals.

Just the facts

- Raloxifene, an osteoporosis-specific designer estrogen, delivers bone protection without increasing the risk of certain cancers.

- SERMs (Selective Estrogen Receptor Modulators) are a new class of lab-designed estrogens for specific uses in the body.

- Tamoxifen is a SERM that protects well against breast cancer.

- More SERMs are in development for potential use in preventing osteoporosis, breast cancer, and other conditions for which postmenopausal women are at risk.

- Nonhormonal medications to treat osteoporosis and overactive bladders are now available.

Treating Menopausal Problems: Beyond Hormones

PART IV

GET THE SCOOP ON...
Vitamins and hot flashes ▪ Increased nutrition
needs during perimenopause and menopause ▪
Nutrients and your moods ▪ Help for
heavy bleeding

Nutrition News

E ating a range of healthy, nutrient-rich foods should help you feel at your best. But while, "you are what you eat" has some basis in truth, it's not as simple as it sounds. Used judiciously, rather than fats necessarily adding fat to your body, some of them keep your system running like a well-oiled machine; without them, in fact, you can't expect much help from your hormones.

The science of nutrition has come a long way from the idea of the Basic Food Groups, which the U.S. government introduced in 1956. We know now about vitamins that weren't thought to exist then and about how certain foods affect moods, for example. Remember when researchers said that butter was bad for you? Now worries about trans-fatty acids, the type of fats found in margarine, are swinging the bread-spread pendulum back in favor of butter as possibly being *better* than margarine. Like the science of everything else, the science of nutrition is still evolving.

Chapter 10

This chapter updates you on the most recent findings that can help your health, and tells you why the suggested daily allowances of many nutrients have been revised upward. In addition, the chapter targets your individual perimenopause and menopause concerns with specific nutritional therapy that has a scientific base. You may be pleasantly surprised by just how much nutrition can help.

Numerous scientific studies show that certain foods can help prevent cancer, aging, and heart disease through their antioxidant actions. Most damage to the body is thought to result from free radicals, highly reactive molecules that can wreak havoc in the body by damaging cell membranes and DNA.

Free radicals are produced in several ways. The most common is simply oxidation, the normal process in which the body breaks down energy. Sometimes in the course of normal oxidation highly charged oxygen molecules (free radicals) are formed. Other times, free radicals are formed by high energy sources (such as X-rays and ultraviolet light) or toxins (such as cigarette smoke). The free radicals formed by these processes are capable of damaging the body's cells. Damage caused by free radicals sets the stage for cancer, blood vessel alterations that result in heart disease, and aging. Antioxidants are compounds capable of neutralizing the effects of these dangerous free radical molecules. Vitamins with these protective capabilities are vitamins A, C, and E. Since fruits and vegetables are rich in these nutrients, the American Cancer Society's recommendation of a minimum of five fruits or vegetables per day seems wise.

Nutrition basics

The U.S. Department of Agriculture's 1995 dietary guidelines include these words to the wise:

- Eat a variety of foods.

- Balance the food that you eat with physical activity to maintain or improve your weight.

- Choose a diet that contains plenty of grain products, vegetables, and fruits.

- Choose a diet that is low in fat, saturated fat, and cholesterol.

- Choose a diet that is moderate in sugars.

- Choose a diet that is moderate in salt and sodium.

- If you drink alcoholic beverages, do so in moderation.

Ideally, nutrition experts say, you should get most of your calories from grain products, vegetables, fruits, low-fat milk products, lean meats, fish, poultry, and dry beans, with fewer calories coming from fats and sweets.

RDAs and RDIs

An apple a day may help keep the doctor away for someone in your household, but for you (or perhaps for your husband or daughter), greater or lesser amounts of nutrients may be necessary. We're all individuals, even in our nutritional requirements.

In the early 1970s the government set U.S. RDAs, or *U.S. Recommended Dietary Allowances*, of nutrients that should be eaten to support health— daily averages representing the amounts of essential nutrients considered adequate to meet the nutritional needs of most healthy persons in the United States.

Bright Idea
Because water-soluble vitamins, such as the Bs and C, can wash out of your body, try to replenish them daily. Good sources of C include citrus fruits and greens. Meats, nuts, and whole grains provide B vitamins. Your body can store fat-soluble vitamins such as A, D, E, and K, so getting them every day isn't as crucial.

There's actually a bit of history to explain behind the term. The U.S. RDA was introduced by the FDA in 1973 as a reference value for vitamins, minerals and protein to be used in voluntary nutrition labeling. But there was some name confusion since the FDA figured its amounts using RDAs (Recommended Dietary Allowances) determined by the National Academy of Sciences.

To distinguish the two, and in the light of expanding scientific understanding about nutrients, the FDA changed its official term from U.S. RDA to RDI (Reference Daily Intake), at the time leaving the actual values the same as the old U.S. RDAs. There's another term you may see also—DRI, or Dietary Reference Intake, a generic term that can encompass other reference values such as the RDA and tolerable upper intake levels.

The National Academy of Sciences' definition of Dietary Reference Intakes includes:

- Recommended Dietary Allowance (RDA): The intake that meets the nutrient need of almost all of the healthy individuals in a specific age and gender group. The RDA should be used in guiding individuals to achieve adequate nutrient intake aimed at decreasing the risk of chronic disease. It is based on estimating an average requirement plus an increase to account for the variation within a particular group.

- Adequate Intake (AI): When sufficient scientific evidence is not available to estimate an average requirement, Adequate Intakes (AIs) have been set. Individuals should use the AI as a goal for intake where no RDAs exist. The AI is derived though experimental or observational data that show a mean intake which appears to sustain a desired indicator of health.

- Estimated Average Requirement (EAR): The intake that meets the estimated nutrient need of half the individuals in a specific group. This figure is to be used as the basis for developing the RDA and is to be used by nutrition policymakers in the evaluation of the adequacy of nutrient intakes of the group and for planning how much the group should consume.

- Tolerable Upper Intake Level (UL): The maximum intake by an individual that is unlikely to pose risks of adverse health effects in almost all healthy individuals in a specified group. This figure is not intended to be a recommended level of intake, and there is no established benefit for individuals to consume nutrients at levels above the RDA or AI.

Nutrition knowledge is by no means static. It has been projected that the entire set of nutrients will be reviewed and Dietary Reference Intakes (DRIs) released by the year 2000, at a research cost of more than 5 million dollars. It's important that along with other dietary recommendations, maximum level guidelines are part of the plan, an effort to reduce risk of adverse health effects from too much of a nutrient.

The sweeping nutrient review is underway a section at a time. Reports have already been issued on DRIs for calcium and its related nutrients phosphorus, magnesium, vitamin D and fluoride, and also for folate, the B vitamins and choline. Still to come are research reports on antioxidants, macronutrients, trace elements, electrolytes, water, and other food components.

Timesaver
You can find answers to basic questions about nutrition at the USDA's Food and Nutrition Information Center Web site at http://www.nal.usda.gov/fnic/ and at the American Dietetic Association's site at www.eatright.org.

New recommendations on calcium, phosphorus, vitamin D, magnesium and fluoride

To decrease the chances of chronic disease, Americans at risk of osteoporosis should consume between 1,000 and 1,300 milligrams of calcium per day (about 1,200 milligrams for those over age 50), according to the Institute of Medicine (National Academy of Sciences) report. Many people don't take in as much as they should. Since bones that are calcium-rich are known to be less susceptible to fractures, the calcium recommendations were set at levels associated with maximum retention of calcium by the body. Tolerable Upper Intake Levels (ULs) were set at 2.5 grams daily for adults.

Other nutrients important to bones were also reviewed, such as phosphorus, so common in many foods that deficiencies are unlikely short of a metabolic disorder or semi-starvation. In order to support normal bone growth and metabolism at various ages, the report recommends a daily intake of about 700 milligrams a day for adults. The Tolerable Upper Intake Level (UL) is 4 grams daily for adults up to age 70, and 3 grams daily for those over 70 years old.

Magnesium interacts with enzymes to regulate body temperature, allow the contraction of muscles and nerves, and make proteins. Recommended intake levels have been revised somewhat upward, though they are not substantially different from the most recent RDAs. About 320 milligrams daily is recommended for women over 30, and a Tolerable Upper Intake Level (UL) is set at 350 milligrams per day of supplemented magnesium (not referring to magnesium from dietary or water sources).

A deficiency of vitamin D can make osteoporosis and other bone problems worse. The vitamin D used

Watch Out!
Pregnant women and nursing mothers may have different nutritional requirements than those described here, as may other population groups whose nutritional requirements are not specifically discussed.

by the body comes mostly through exposure to the sun (it is absorbed through the skin), and newly recommended intake levels are estimated to provide enough even for those who get only limited sun exposure. These recommended levels are higher than levels recommended in earlier RDAs for people over 50. Rather than an RDA, an Adequate Intake (AI) level has been established (see the definition of AIs earlier in this chapter). It is 5 micrograms daily for those age 50 and under, 10 micrograms for those aged 51 to 70, and 15 micrograms for those over 70 years of age. The Tolerable Upper Intake (UL) is set at 50 micrograms daily.

In many water systems where fluoride isn't naturally present, it is added in order to reduce tooth decay. DRI recommendations set a level of intake (Adequate Intake of 3.1 milligrams a day for adults) shown to reduce dental decay without causing marked fluorosis (a discoloring of the teeth that can occur with overuse of fluoride). The Tolerable Upper Intake Level (UL) was set at 10 milligrams a day.

A fresh look at the B vitamins and their safety

Another 1998 report from the Institute of Medicine (National Academy of Sciences) reviews the need for the B vitamins (including folate) and choline. Women of childbearing age are now recommended to take in 400 micrograms of folate daily, which is about twice what American women do consume, and significantly more than the longstanding RDA of 180 micrograms a day. Folate is a nutrient (considered among the B vitamins) that helps prevent birth defects, aids in the development of red blood cells and may help protect against heart disease. You'll find it in leafy vegetables, lentils, orange juice and other foods, and since 1998 it has been added

Unofficially...
To best set vitamin D intake recommendations, researchers are interested in exploring the effects of sunscreen on vitamin D absorption from sunlight.

Unofficially...
How about a diet including triple-boiled green beans, carrots, chicken, turkey or ham for weeks? Ten postmenopausal women in San Francisco already tried this for science. The U.S. Agricultural Research Service study they were in yielded new information about how much women need folate, a B vitamin. This research added to evidence for increasing the old RDA of folate for women.

to enriched grain products (such as pasta and cereals) sold in the United States. Folic acid is the synthetic form of folate and is used in supplements.

Except for folate, most of the recommendations for B vitamins are similar to old RDAs, and most Americans meet their requirements through their diet. And while much research in the past twenty years has looked at how B vitamins may reduce the risk of cardiovascular disease, cancers or various psychiatric or mental disorders, it is not considered a solid enough body of evidence to base nutritional recommendations on (however, the Institute of Medicine report considers this research provocative). The new guidelines for B intakes are instead based on values shown to guard against anemia or other vitamin deficiency ailments.

Beyond folate, recommendations for adult women are as follows:

- Thiamin: 1.1 milligrams

- Riboflavin: 1.1 milligrams

- Niacin: 14 milligrams

- B_6: 1.3 milligrams (1.5 for women over 30)

- B_{12}: 2.4 micrograms

- Panthothenic acid: 5 milligrams (Adequate Intake Level)

- Biotin: 30 micrograms (Adequate Intake Level)

- Choline: 425 milligrams (Adquate Intake Level)

Some of the most interesting recommendations in the report have to do with Tolerable Upper Intake Limits (ULs). For vitamin B_6, this is set at 100 milligrams per day for adults. Above that amount, intake could cause sensory neuropathy (a nerve disorder that can lead to pain, numbness, and weakness in the limbs). Too much folic acid can put individuals who have a B_{12} deficiency at greater risk of progressive, crippling neurologic damage, so a folate UL of 1,000 micrograms (1 milligram) was set for adults. Too much niacin can result in the well-known niacin flush, with warm sensation and itching among other symptoms, so an upper limit was set at 35 milligrams per day. A Tolerable Upper Intake Level for choline is now set at 3.5 grams per day for adults since above that level low blood pressure may result, as well as a fishy body odor in some people.

Researchers looking into safe levels of other B vitamins cited a lack of studies on adverse effects at higher intake ranges. Because of it they did not set upper limits for thiamin, riboflavin, vitamin B_{12}, pantothenic acid, and biotin. But they did urge extra caution about overconsumption since so little data is available.

Antioxidant avengers

Numerous scientific studies show that certain foods can help prevent cancer, aging, and heart disease through their antioxidant actions. Most damage to the body is thought to result from free radicals, highly reactive molecules that can wreak havoc in the body by damaging cell membranes and DNA.

Free radicals are produced in several ways. The most common is simply, oxidation, the normal process in which the body breaks down energy. Sometimes in the course of normal oxidation highly charged oxygen molecules (free radicals) are formed. Other times, free radicals are formed by high energy sources (such as X-rays and ultraviolet light) or toxins (such as cigarette smoke). The free radicals formed by these processes are capable of damaging the body's cells. Damage caused by free radicals sets the stage for cancer, blood vessels

Watch Out!
Since up to 30 percent of older people may mal-absorb food-bound B_{12}, it's advisable for those over 50 to meet their RDA from foods forti-fied with B_{12} or a B_{12}-containing supplement.

Watch Out!
If you already take a high-dose niacin supple-ment, you may be exceeding the Tolerable Upper Intake Limit for niacin (35 mil-ligrams daily).

Watch Out!
Think a vitamin/mineral pill will give you everything you need? Think again. Nutrition experts favor food over supplements because food naturally has an array of other lesser-known nutrients, such as phytochemicals, whose actions may be of great help to the body.

alterations that result in heart disease, and aging. Antioxidants are compounds capable of neutralizing the effects of these dangerous free radical molecules. Vitamins with these protective capabilities are vitamins A, C, and E. Since fruits and vegetables are rich in these nutrients, the American Cancer Society's recommendation of a minimum of five fruits or vegetables per day seems wise.

A balance of nutrients is, of course, necessary for good health. Many supplements contain far higher levels of various nutrients than the RDAs, because some believe they *may* more profoundly support good health. As described earlier in this chapter, however, it is wise to be careful of the dangers inherent in oversupplementing. In coming years guidelines for Tolerable Upper Intake Levels on a wider variety of nutrients should help consumers sort out when it's really safe to take a supplement—and when it's not. Water-soluble vitamins mix with water and are easily excreted, which makes them less likely to accumulate in toxic levels. Conversely, fat-soluble vitamins (A, D, E and K) do not mix with water, are not easily excreted, and may be stored in fat deposits in the body. Taking excessive doses of these types of vitamins, especially vitamins A and D can lead to toxic levels with adverse effects.

Putting it all together

How much of the various nutrients do you need? Table 10.1 shows the amounts recommended by the National Academy of Sciences for adult women, incorporating the recently reviewed nutrient levels. It is a potent antioxidant. But excess levels should be avoided as vitamin A can easily be toxic to the liver and cause other very serious problems in high enough doses.

TABLE 10.1: RECOMMENDED DIETARY ALLOWANCES (FOR WOMEN AGE 19 TO 50/ unless otherwise stated)

Nutrient	Amount
Vitamins	
A	800 micrograms
D	5 micrograms (through age 50) 10 micrograms (age 51 to 70) 15 micrograms (age 70 and above)
E	8 milligrams
K	60 micrograms (age 19 to 24) 65 micrograms (age 25 to 50)
C	60 milligrams
Thiamin (B_1)	1.1 milligrams
Riboflavin (B_2)	1.1 milligrams
Niacin (B_3)	14 milligrams
Pyridoxine (B_6)	1.5 milligrams (women over 30)
Folate	400 micrograms
Cobalmin (B_{12})	2.4 micrograms
Minerals	
Calcium	1,000 milligrams (age 50 and under) 1,200 milligrams (over age 50)
Phosphorus	700 milligrams
Magnesium	320 milligrams (women over 30)
Iron	15 milligrams
Zinc	12 milligrams
Iodine	150 micrograms
Selenium	55 micrograms

Vital Vitamins

Vitamins and minerals act synergistically in the body to sustain life. They are as necessary as hormones themselves, and some vitamins actually *are* hormones.

Beta-carotene

Your body can turn beta-carotene into vitamin A as needed, without the same toxicity posed by high doses of vitamin A. Good blood levels of beta-carotene have been associated with less risk of certain cancers than low blood levels of beta-carotene. Research is continuing on the potential benefits, but *it* may not be without risks either. An extensive Finnish research study designed to find out if beta-carotene might help protect against lung cancer instead found a *higher* risk of lung and other cancers in smoking men aged 50 and older who used it (at doses of 20mg per day, a level analogous to more than triple the RDA of vitamin A). It is not the only study to have found an increased risk of lung cancer in smokers who took supplemental beta-carotene, and other research casts doubt on the idea that beta-carotene might protect against cardiovascular disease. High dosages of beta carotene can turn your skin yellowish. Reducing intake of foods rich in vitamin A, such as carrots, reverses this situation.

Vitamin B₁ (thiamin)

The main duty of Vitamin B_1 (also called *thiamin*) involves metabolism, the breakdown of food components into energy. The vitamin helps to maintain the nervous system, heart, and muscular tissue.

Vitamin B₂ (riboflavin)

Vitamin B_2 (riboflavin) also aids in metabolism. It's crucial to the formation of red blood cells and benefits your immune system, not to mention maintaining healthy eyes and hair.

Vitamin B₃ (niacin)

Vitamin B_3 (niacin) is another vitamin that is necessary for metabolism of fats, proteins, and carbohydrates. It helps to lower cholesterol, and may be useful in depression and insomnia At very high doses it

Watch Out!
Niacin, taken in high dosage, can cause facial flushing and heat not dissimilar to hot flashes. During menopause, you may be more comfortable taking a specially formulated, non-flushing type of niacin that prevents this reaction. It is available as a supplement and sometimes is included in multiple vitamins.

can have serious side effects, including high blood sugar, liver damage and irregular heartbeat, and even at levels only a few times the RDA, niacin can cause flushing and other discomforts.

Vitamin B$_5$ (pantothenic acid)

Vitamin B$_5$ (pantothenic acid) helps regulate the body's use of energy and helps it use other vitamins. This vitamin is important in regulating your body's response to stress and in ensuring smooth functioning of the nervous system and adrenal glands.

Vitamin B$_6$ (pyridoxine)

Vitamin B$_6$ (pyridoxine) is active in metabolism, particularly of protein. The vitamin also helps regulate the nervous system. Although widely touted as a remedy to relieve water retention associated with premenstrual syndrome (PMS), this claim has not been duplicated in the medical literature. Toxic reactions, including loss of sensation in the hands and feet, have occurred when women took megadoses of this vitamin (400 times the RDA) to relieve PMS symptoms. Luckily these reactions are reversible when dosages are decreased.

Vitamin B$_{12}$ (cobalmin)

Vitamin B$_{12}$ is essential in the making of red blood cells, and like iron, it is necessary to prevent anemia. It is necessary for the proper function of the nervous system and helps in metabolism and calcium absorption as well. Cobalmin is present in meat, fish, eggs, and milk. Strict vegetarians (and some people with gastrointestinal disorders who are thus incapable of absorbing this vitamin) may need supplementation. It can be given as an injection, sublingual lozenge, or nasal spray.

Vitamin C (ascorbic acid)

Vitamin C is crucial to your bones, teeth, gums, and a host of other tissues. It is a major antioxidant, countering damage from pollution and other toxins, and it figures prominently in wound healing. Vitamin C may help prevent cancer as well.

Vitamin D (calciferol)

Vitamin D is necessary for the body's proper use of calcium and other minerals; therefore, it figures prominently in the maintenance of healthy bones (teeth and gums, too). It also helps keep your nervous system and cardiovascular system healthy. But levels significantly in excess of those recommended can be hard on the kidneys and may cause other health problems.

Vitamin E (tocopherol)

Vitamin E is another important antioxidant, countering damage to cells by neutralizing dangerous free radicals. The vitamin may also alleviate tiredness, hot flashes, and vaginal dryness; improve mood; and thin the blood. Vitamin E is used to ensure cardiac and brain health, particularly after certain kinds of strokes or heart attacks, and is also used to prevent those disorders.

Biotin and folic acid

Biotin and folic acid are particularly important for healthy hair and nails. The latter also figures in the growth of all body cells. A deficiency of folic acid can be responsible for prematurely graying hair. The recommended daily intake guidelines were recently modified to reflect higher folic acid levels following research suggesting folic acid may help during pregnancy to prevent spinal cord birth defects.

Unofficially... PABA (para-amino-benzoic-acid) is a nutrient that you may know best as a sunscreen. PABA deficiency can produce fatigue and skin problems, along with graying hair.

Inositol and choline

Inositol helps prevent hair thinning, aids in the metabolization of fats, and can reduce cholesterol. Choline is important in this regard as well, and also facilitates memory and nerve transmission.

Meaningful minerals

Minerals are just as important to your body as vitamins are, and you can't make minerals on your own. The following sections describe the vital functions of various minerals.

Calcium

Calcium is important for the bones, teeth, and heart. It can help insomnia as well. Calcium figures in nerve function; it also lowers blood pressure and cholesterol, and counters muscle cramps. A deficiency can lead to osteoporosis.

Magnesium

Magnesium is important for proper heart function, as well as for the proper use of calcium by the body and the conversion of sugars to energy.

Iron

Iron is crucial for making red blood cells, providing oxygen to the tissues, and preventing anemia and fatigue, as well as for fostering immunity. Too much is dangerous to the kidneys, liver, and heart.

Iodine

A deficiency in iodine can lead to major thyroid problems, which is why iodine is added to most brands of table salt. Iodine is also crucial for helping the body produce energy. A sluggish metabolism can mean too little iodine or the inability to use it properly.

Watch Out!
Don't get too much of a good thing. Think carefully before deciding to supplement vitamins or minerals at levels much above the RDAs, and discuss your intended supplement with your physician. Extra care is needed to avoid exacerbating certain health conditions.

Watch Out!
If you get constipation or stomach upset from regular iron supplements, try a more easily absorbed time-released version.

Copper

Copper helps the body properly metabolize iron and use vitamin C. The mineral also helps the body build bone and form red blood cells, among other things.

Zinc

Zinc is necessary for proper maintenance of the reproductive system and for wound healing. Zinc is also an antioxidant, and in some studies, it has been found to help reduce the duration of the common cold.

Manganese

Manganese works with copper and zinc to promote bone growth. It also helps to maintain muscles and nerves. Since manganese is naturally obtained from red meat, vegetarians are at increased risk of deficiency and potentially weak bones.

Unofficially...
Niacin has been found to improve cholesterol levels and decrease homocysteine levels, and is becoming very important in treating coronary artery disease.

Fluoride

It's been recognized for some time that the addition of fluoride to water promotes strong, healthy teeth. Fluoride is also essential to strong bone formation, and supplements can help deter osteoporosis.

Treat yourself

As more research has been done on nutritional supplements' beneficial effects on several conditions, doctors have increasingly begun to prescribe specific vitamins and minerals almost as though they were drugs, when reliable study results clearly indicate that those compounds can help.

Such is the case for some difficulties that women experience during perimenopause and menopause. Vitamin E, for example, has been touted as an anecdote for hot flashes, although a recent study found only a minimal reduction in number of flashes. There was no apparent toxicity to the treatment.

What other specific nutrients can help you in a menopausal tight spot? Beyond ensuring that you get enough vitamins, minerals, and other nutrients, you can target specific problems with nutritional therapy. Tables 10.2 and 10.3 provide a guide to what's good for what.

TABLE 10.2: NUTRIENTS FOR MENOPAUSAL SYMPTOMS

Symptoms	Nutrients
Excessive bleeding	Iron (to prevent anemia), protein, vitamin C
Hot flashes	Vitamin E
Mood swings and stress	Vitamin E, B vitamins

TABLE 10.3: NUTRIENTS FOR POSTMENOPAUSAL CONDITIONS

Condition	Nutrients
Alzheimer's disease	Vitamin E, phosphytydalserine
Heart disease	Vitamin E (also vitamin C and other antioxidants, magnesium, CoQ 10, taurine, niacin)
Osteoporosis	Calcium, vitamin D, folic acid, copper, zinc, manganese, flouride, magnesium, silicon, boron and various amino acids

← **Note!**
Phosphatidylserine is a phospholipid nutrient found in cell membranes and can be derived from lecithin. Preliminary research has associated it with improvements in memory and overall decrease in dementia in Alzheimer's patients.

Heads, hearts, and hot flashes

The benefits of vitamin E are becoming increasingly well known. Vitamin E is a powerful antioxidant that can help repair damaged tissue and prevent heart attacks. It even figures in stroke recovery and treatment of Alzheimer's disease—such is its powerful effect in the brain. For women who are grappling with perimenopause or menopause, vitamin E is a

Unofficially...
You may see the name *tocopherol* associated with vitamin E. The word originated from the words *tokos* (for *childbirth*) and *pherein* (meaning *to bring forth*), with *ol* stuck on to signify the chemical structure phenol. Vitamin E is made up of a few types of tocopherol and a few types of tocotrienol.

potential defense for hot flashes and for some of the symptoms that go with them, such as sweating mood swings.

As far as the vasomotor instability known as hot flashes is concerned, *vitamin E* might help. Multiple studies half a century ago and anecdotal reports today support the use of vitamin E in alleviating hot flashes and helping with other difficulties in menopause, such as vaginal dryness. One 1949 entry in the *British Medical Journal* noted that vitamin E relieved severe menopausal flushing in 64 percent of patients studied (at 500 international units a day—a high dose). Research focusing on vitamin E's uses in menopause fell out of the limelight in decades that followed, however, as estrogen came on the scene.

Today, interest in vitamin E's potential benefits to menopausal women is again picking up, though a recent study published in the *Journal of Clinical Oncology* was not able to duplicate the earlier-reported benefits of vitamin E for hot flashes, when tested in breast cancer survivors. Although 800 milligrams daily of vitamin E did appear to reduce the number of hot flashes experienced by test subjects, it was a marginal reduction.

Even though vitamin E is a fat soluble vitamin that can accumulate in the body, it has a relatively low toxicity profile. Potential toxic reactions include a decrease in white blood cells (the segment of blood cells that fight infection), liver dysfunction, and interference with blood coagulation. When taken in high doses, it may also raise blood pressure.

You can get vitamin E in your diet from some vegetable oils, as well as nuts and seeds. As a supplement, vitamin E is often contained in good dosages in multiple vitamins. Seek vitamin E from a natural rather than synthetic source. Mixed tocopherols mentioned somewhere on the bottle are a good sign of a complete E supplement. New forms of E are now available, such as dry E (d-alpha tocopheryl succinate) and water-soluble E, for increased absorption.

Because vitamin E can make anticoagulant medications even more potent, discuss the use of vitamin E with your doctor if you're taking anticoagulants (such as coumadin) or even daily aspirin. The use of vitamin E before surgery is often discouraged for the same reason, although the vitamin may help you heal later. It's also wise to review your medical history with your doctor before taking particularly high doses of vitamin E—more than 600 IU daily, for example. Finally, be sure to add other antioxidants to your daily diet or supplement program. Vitamin E works synergistically with different nutrients, such as vitamin C, and the benefits that you get are likely to be more dramatic.

Vitamin E can help prevent atherosclerosis (hardening of the arteries) and heart problems, and can help regulate cholesterol levels by reducing LDL, the bad cholesterol. A well-known Nurses' Health Study tracked more than 87,000 women ages 34 to 59 for several years, and found that vitamin E figured into reduced levels of cardiac disease. Interestingly, risk reduction required taking vitamin E supplements for at least two years. By decreasing clot formation vitamin E shows promise in decreasing the risk of heart attacks and strokes. While the RDA for vitamin E is 8 milligrams, (which corresponds to 12 IU) vitamin E benefits mentioned above require larger doses. Most authorities feel a

Timesaver
The newer measurement of vitamin E is in milligrams (mg) rather than the out of date International Units (IU). Reference to IU is common, especially when previous research is quoted. The conversion is as follows:

10 mg = 15 IU

To convert mg to IU, multiply the number of milligrams by 1.5. To convert IU to mg, multiply the number of IU by 0.6.

beneficial dose that avoids potential toxicity is 400 IU (equivalent to 266 milligrams). Antioxidant benefits of vitamin E are being actively investigated.

Although vitamin E can work more quickly in stemming the incidence of hot flashes, you should take it consistently and long term to gain its other benefits.

The value of vitamin A

Although a full range of nutrients is necessary for proper endocrine health and reproductive function, different ones play different roles. Vitamin A, for example, was found in one study to resolve vaginal yeast infections. Women who had suffered frequent infections were found to have lower-than-normal vitamin A levels. And in animal studies, cows that didn't receive enough beta-carotene (which the body turns into vitamin A) had increased rates of infertility, irregular menstruation, and ovarian cysts.

There is often confusion between vitamin A and beta-carotene. They are related by the body's ability to convert beta-carotene to vitamin A. An important point is that vitamin A is fat-soluble while beta-carotene is water-soluble. This means that vitamin A can reach toxic and dangerous levels (roughly 10 times the RDA will result in toxicity), whereas beta-carotene can be more safely ingested (see comments earlier in this chapter, however, about the potential risks of beta-carotene). Both sources deliver healthy antioxidant effects, with most of the benefit in vitamin supplements coming from beta-carotene because of relative safety. Good dietary sources of vitamin A include milk, liver, butter, and eggs (animal origin). Good dietary sources of beta-carotene include carrots, green leafy vegetables, cantaloupe, and broccoli (plant origin).

Watch Out!
Be careful about taking too much vitamin A, since the potential for side effects is high. Toxic levels can result in headache, vision disturbance, skin rash, hair loss, and insomnia. Excessive dosages have been linked to liver and brain damage. (If too much vitamin A is taken in early pregnancy, birth defects can occur.

The beneficial Bs

The B vitamins are often called stress vitamins, and their use is associated with maintaining good energy levels. B vitamins should generally be taken in a balanced form, containing the entire range of Bs. Vitamin B_6 (pyridoxine) may reduce water retention in PMS. B_6 is also involved in the development of neurotransmitters, so deficiencies may result in anxiety or depression. It makes sense to get adequate amounts of these vitamins in your diet, especially during menopause when emotional changes can occur.

Good food sources of the B vitamins include bananas, potatoes, whole grains, nuts, and seeds.

You can find even more mood support in a diet that is low in refined carbohydrates (such as sugar, processed breads, and processed cereals), not excessive in fat, and high in foods that pack a big nutrient punch. Go for whole grains, fresh vegetables and fruits, legumes, and lean meats. And make sure to eat adequate protein and complex carbohydrates early in the day so that you'll have sustained energy.

Skeletal support

Bone strength requires certain building blocks: calcium, vitamins A and D, trace elements (such as copper, zinc, and manganese), as well as phosphorus. Calcium and vitamin D are essential to proper bone function; a lack of these nutrients can encourage osteoporosis. Many studies have affirmed the role of adequate calcium supplementation in staving off bone loss. A long-term study of postmenopausal women, reported in the *New England Journal of Medicine* (1993), compared a control group ingesting an average 750 milligrams of calcium daily with a group that got 1,000 milligrams

TimeSaver
Vitamin A and beta-carotene are sure to be important players in future studies and nutrition due to their antioxidant properties. Newer terminology for these compounds measures vitamin A activity in terms of retinol equivalents (RE). The following conversions are used:

1 RE = 1 microgram (mcg) retinol (the form of vitamin a in animal products) = 6 micrograms (mcg) beta-carotene

Bright Idea
Because caffeine causes the body to secrete stress hormones, cutting back on it (as well as simple carbohydrates and alcohol) can often alleviate anxiety and depression after just a short time.

Bright Idea
There's an easy way to test your calcium supplement's ability to get absorbed by your body. Cover the pill with distilled white vinegar and observe it over the course of the next half-hour. If it fails to dissolve in that period of time it will not dissolve properly in your body and will therefore not deliver its full dose to you. You may want to choose another supplement.

more calcium via a daily supplement. Calcium supplementation had a beneficial effect on bone loss. The placebo group lost bone at a rate of about 1 percent a year, but that loss was reduced by almost half in the group that received extra calcium.

Most women cannot get adequate calcium in their diet alone, so calcium supplements are needed. There are many different types on the market. Calcium carbonate has the highest percentage of available calcium and is the most commonly used supplement, but it is poorly absorbed by the body. Side effects include constipation, bloating, and gas. Calcium citrate is more easily absorbed by the stomach although it supplies less calcium per tablet. This form is sometimes added to orange juice. Look for this in your supermarket since it is an "easy to swallow" form of calcium with fewer side effects. Antacids such as Tums and Rolaids contain calcium carbonate. They are readily available and relieve heartburn as well. In older women there is often a reduced ability to absorb nutrients like calcium due to low levels of hydrochloric acid in the stomach. For them, calcium citrate is the better choice, as it is easily absorbed regardless of stomach acid levels.

Be careful not to overdo it when taking calcium supplements. Side effects include constipation, bloating, interference with absorption of other minerals such as iron and zinc, interference with absorption of medications such as tetracycline, some antidiabetic and anticonvulsant medications, and potential exacerbation of kidney stones in susceptible people. The best approach is to get as much calcium as possible from dietary sources with supplements used to make up the difference.

People who are lactose intolerant can get calcium from nonmilk products such as spinach, tofu, beans, and green vegetables. Lactose-free milk is another good option. There are certain foods that can decrease calcium availability. Caffeine and animal protein promote excretion via the kidneys. Alcohol, carbonated beverages, large amounts of fiber, and foods high in oxalates (compounds found in spinach, rhubarb, and chocolate) decrease absorption from the gut. Taking your supplement shortly after eating a meal or snack is a good idea since the stomach acids used to digest food aid the absorption of calcium as well.

Vitamin D can promote calcium absorption and help further prevent osteoporosis.

Calcium sources include dairy products, which are often fortified. Fish (such as salmon), tofu, and certain vegetables and legumes (broccoli, peas, beans, and lettuces such as arugula) are good sources, too. Seeds, nuts, and whole grains also provide calcium.

There are other nutrients that are important to keep bones strong. Folic acid and adequate B vitamins (particularly B_6) are needed to prevent osteoporosis. Copper is also necessary for good bone health; a deficiency of copper can lead to weakened bones and anemia. Excess of copper can cause other serious problems, however. Schizophrenia, learning disabilities, and senility are among the conditions being investigated for potential links to excess copper levels. Many nutritionists do not supplement copper because of toxicity concerns (and at least not more than 2 mg a day, the RDA for adults).

You can get copper in your diet from seafood, organ meats, most dried beans, grains, and nuts. If you have copper water pipes or use copper pans to

Bright Idea
Don't wait until you're through menopause to add a calcium supplement. The most important time to get a sufficient amount is while your bones are still consolidating during early and middle adulthood. Building solid bones earlier can help prevent fractures later . . . bone up!

Timesaver
Don't confuse the amount of elemental calcium (the amount of calcium in the tablet) with total compound weight. For example, Tums E-X contains 750 mg of calcium carbonate (the total compound) and 300 mg of elemental calcium.

Bright Idea
Don't wait until you're through menopause to add a calcium supplement. The most important time to get a sufficient amount is while your bones are still consolidating during early and middle adulthood. Building solid bones earlier can help prevent fractures later . . . bone up!

cook with, you may be getting additional copper from those sources.

Iron woman

The RDA for iron in adult women is 15 milligrams daily—5 milligrams more than men should have. Women need more iron because they can lose 15 to 20 milligrams in blood loss during each period. Without enough iron, you can become anemic. Signs of iron-deficiency anemia include paleness, headaches, and fatigue. Adequate protein is also necessary during excessive bleeding.

Good sources of iron include some of the same sources recommended for protein: meat, fish, and poultry. Peas and beans, spinach and other green leafy vegetables, potatoes, and whole-grain and iron-fortified cereal products also provide iron, although of a type that is not as easily absorbed as iron from animal sources. Vitamin C has also been reported to help restore balance when heavy bleeding is present. Whenever possible try to eat a food rich in vitamin C in conjunction with iron-rich food since vitamin C increases the body's ability to absorb iron. Be careful of ingesting excessive amounts of iron supplements, however. Iron toxicity can occur, especially in menopausal women who no longer bleed. These effects include arthritis, diabetes, and liver damage. A genetics-linked disorder called hemochromatosis can double the amount of iron a person absorbs. Excess iron may not be noticed for many years until it accumulates and starts to damage organs (some symptoms include frequent urination, fatigue, and persistent thirst). There is some research to show a serious excess of iron *may* also be implicated in the development of breast and colon cancers.

Amino acids: Mood foods and more

Amino acids are components of protein that help build your body. Along with repairing tissue and completing a host of other functions, these nutrients are crucial to the functioning of your hormones.

There are 22 known amino acids, 8 of which are considered to be essential in the diet because they can't be manufactured by the body. These essential amino acids are as follows:

- Tryptophan

- Lysine

- Methionine

- Phenylalanine

- Threonine

- Valine

- Leucine

- Isoleucine

You can choose foods that are high in certain amino acids to elicit the effects that you want, or you can take specific amino-acid supplements for many of them.

Tryptophan, for example, can actually be a sedative. If you've ever felt sleepy after eating a turkey dinner at Thanksgiving, that situation *may* have been due to the high amounts of tryptophan in turkey. Consider using tryptophan-rich foods to help curb insomnia. Tryptophan can also help reduce anxiety, alleviate depression, and treat migraine headaches. Foods containing lots of tryptophan include turkey and other fowl, yogurt and unripened cheese, pineapple and bananas.

Lysine helps you absorb calcium and aids in hormonal production and regulation. Women

Unofficially...
After menopause, a woman's iron stores gradually increase, and iron-deficiency anemia is less likely to occur.

who have deficiencies may develop anemia and reproductive difficulties. Deficiencies can result in lethargy, irritability, difficulty concentrating, and hair loss. You'll find lysine in fish, lean meat, milk, and potatoes.

Methionine is particularly important for skin, nails, and hair. It can also promote healthy liver function and reduce cholesterol levels. It can be helpful in cases of fatigue and as an allergy reducer since it reduces the release of histamine. It may also help tremors in Parkinson's disease. Common sources include meats, eggs, cottage cheese, yogurt, soybeans, sardines, and lentils.

Phenylalanine is an important brain precursor to norepinephrine, which is a key neurotransmitter. Norepinephrine is largely responsible for alertness; it can help alleviate depression, increase focus, and boost memory. Norepinephrine stores can be depleted when you've been up to your ears in stress, too, so adequate phenylalanine intake is especially important. It is present in cheese and meat.

Valine figures both in calming emotional distress and in stimulating mental alertness and muscular coordination. Therefore, it is also an important stress amino acid. Some valine sources are cottage cheese, meat, nuts, chickpeas and mushrooms.

Leucine and *isoleucine* are necessary for the body to create energy and support brain function and alertness. Meat and dairy products are chief sources.

Other amino acids are considered to be nonessential, although some are useful for specific purposes. Arginine, tyrosine, glycine, serine, glutamic acid, aspartic acid, taurine, cysteine, histidine, proline, and alanine are all nonessential amino acids, which means that the body can manufacture them from other building blocks.

Arginine is necessary for tissue repair and hormonal regulation, spurring growth-hormone release, among other duties.

Tyrosine is important for thyroid function (as is the mineral iodine), as well as for pituitary and adrenal function. As a result, tyrosine is very important in balancing the hormones and stimulating metabolism for sustenance of the entire body. It can help relieve depression and improve memory as well.

Glutamic acid helps improve mental faculties and can help alleviate lethargy, so it's a good treatment for the fuzzy thinking that sometimes occurs during menopause.

EFAs: Fats you have to have

Striving to include as little fat as possible in your diet is not healthy at all, and meals would be more than a little bland, to boot. Fats, in fact, are essential to survival. The brain is largely made up of components of fat, and cholesterol itself is what your sex hormones are made from. Fat does not necessarily make you fat, either; your body is quite capable of storing carbohydrates and even proteins as fat.

The type of fat that you eat can play a big role in determining your health. All fats are not created equal. *Essential fatty acids* (EFAs) are the crucial building blocks for several body processes, ranging from how we burn fat to the hormones that we make to our moods. There are even good fats that help prevent damage from bad fats—the kind that can lead to excessive cholesterol levels and a wide range of damage.

Two fatty acids that are necessary for survival are *linoleic acid* (also called omega-6) and *alpha-linelenic acid,* (also called omega-3), without which our

Unofficially...
Fat's reputation for encouraging obesity stems from its nature as a calorically dense food. A gram of protein or carbohydrate has 3 to 4 calories, whereas a gram of fat has at least double the caloric value.

bodies can't adequately produce the other fatty acids that it uses. These acids are known as *unsaturated fats,* due to their chemical structure. Deficiencies of the fatty acids can lead to skin and hair problems; liver disease; poor wound healing; miscarriage; retarded growth, vision, and learning ability; arthritis; and heart problems. Some women find that deficiencies also contribute to peri-menopause, encouraging PMS, mood swings, and edema.

Getting adequate quantities of EFAs can often relieve dry skin, improve mental function and body metabolism (plus edema), and reduce high blood pressure and triglycerides.

Following are some of the beneficial oils that you can add to your diet:

- *Flaxseed oil,* which is rich in what are called omega-3 fatty acids and other components that help stabilize estrogen levels.

- *Evening primrose oil,* which may help with emotional symptoms and fluid retention, and which is a rich source of omega-6 oils.

- *Borage and black currant seed oils,* which also supply omega-6 fatty acids.

- *Fish oils,* which are rich sources of omega-3, include sardines, salmon, whitefish, herring, swordfish, tuna, and bass.

There is much scientific interest in these two EFAs. Recent studies suggest key roles for these fats in promoting and preventing disease. Omega-3 fats seem to be the most beneficial, potentially decreasing cancer and heart disease. Large amounts of omega-6 oil, on the other hand, may promote tumor growth. Oils rich in this type of oil are corn and safflower. Oils that contain a balance of omega-6 and omega-3 seem to be beneficial.

Considering cravings

If you've ever seen a pet gnaw on grass for an upset stomach, you know that instinct plays a role in the foods that we choose. Although no one would suggest that this means going whole-hog on sweets (there are such things as pathological cravings), don't be quick to dismiss a monthly yearning for some specific food as being a fault. Many women experience cravings as part of PMS.

Cravings may be all in your head—that is, your body may be calling out for specific neurotransmitter support that is best provided by the food you desire most. If you've had a child, you know that cravings can run rampant during pregnancy, be they for pickles and ice cream or something equally bizarre. At that time, with two people to provide for, your body's not interested in protocol so much as it is in having its needs met on the double. When you think about it, a craving for pickles and ice cream is not that bizarre at all. Pickles supply the salt needed to promote fluid accumulation (our bodies are predominantly made up of water, and salt is necessary to retain that water). Ice-cream supplies the quick demand for carbohydrates (and, therefore, energy).

Before you read up on what specific food cravings can mean, try filling out Worksheet 10.1 to analyze your own cravings.

The foods that you choose may not be just comfort foods or those that provide a fast carbohydrate energy boost. Consider chocolate, which is a frequently craved food. Half of women surveyed actually said that they would choose chocolate over

Unofficially...
As many as half of all women have food cravings when they're pregnant. The foods that pregnant women most frequently obsess about include fruit and fruit juices, sweet foods, and dairy products. Cravings typically are most pronounced during the first trimester.

Note! ➡
Some foods that women typically crave are chocolate and other sweets, red meat, salty and fatty foods, and sometimes—believe it or not—greens.

WORKSHEET 10.1: CHARTING CRAVINGS

List the foods that you typically crave, along with when you want them most, and any specifics (see the example). Then guess what your body is trying to tell you.

Food	Craved When?	Notes	Why?
Chocolate	Premenstrually, when busy and anxious	Dark chocolate, not light	Comfort food
_____	_____	_____	_____
_____	_____	_____	_____
_____	_____	_____	_____
_____	_____	_____	_____

sex, writes Debra Waterhouse in her book *Why Women Need Chocolate* (Hyperion, 1995).

Chocoholics, unite!

Chocolate, like love itself, has the capability to efficiently boost the pleasure centers of our brains through the release of endorphins. A chemical component called phenylethylamine helps provide the high, along with the stimulants caffeine and theobromine. Chocolate has also been found to contain chemicals known as cannabinoids, which are—you guessed it—the active compounds in marijuana (albeit at significantly lower levels).

Particularly if you crave dark, rich chocolate, you may be craving the cocoa-butter component, which provides the fatty acids that are necessary for hormone and neurotransmitter development. Although the sweet taste means simple sugars that can provide quick energy, the fat also means a longer-term source of fuel, which helps buffer the glycemic (blood-sugar) effect and keeps you from experiencing the fatigue that can set in after a simple-sugar high. Both the sweet and fatty portions may boost brain levels of serotonin, the neurotransmitter that is linked to comfort and that figures in a wide range of antidepressant medications.

Chocolate also contains the amino acids phenylalanine and tyrosine, which are important neurotransmitter precursors. Consider the saltiness of chocolate as well; your body may be crying out for mineral support.

Studies of why cravings occur and whether fulfilling them helps have provided contradictory answers. One often-noted study on chocolate found that research subjects were not satisfied when they were given the chemical components of chocolate; the taste, texture, and scent of chocolate were necessary to the experience.

Science is still sorting out answers, so when you're thinking about supplementing nutrients elsewhere in your diet, it may be helpful to remember that the body does not operate in a vacuum. In other words, don't eschew natural whole foods in favor of eating processed foods that have little nutritional value and taking a vitamin/mineral supplement on the side. Given the number of new nutrients that have recently been discovered, you'll more than likely miss out on something necessary or something that's held in balance by the presence of other substances in a particular food. No matter what the futurists of the 1950s thought (about the 1980s, to be exact), we're not about to pop protein pills in favor of real food—pills and food are *not the same thing.*

Unofficially...
Chocolate contains the pheromone (olfactory sexual attractant) dimethyl disulfide. Alas, the only males tested and found to be aroused by the stuff are male rats.

Watch Out!
Feeling a little depressed and wanting chocolate? Give your body a steady supply of complex carbohydrates, which could prevent mood deflation. Or consider taking a good mineral supplement. The jury is still out on the benefit or detriment of chocolate in treating PMS and similar perimenopausal and menopausal problems.

When you have a craving, indulge it, but do so wisely. Half a bar of dark chocolate without a lot of additives may do the trick; it's not necessary to eat an entire box of chocolate cookies. And by going for the concentrated stuff—real chocolate made with real cocoa butter—you stand a better chance of providing the substances that your body's asking for than if you opt for something that's merely chocolate-flavored and fat-free, tricking only your taste buds into thinking that all is well.

You can also use food cravings to alert yourself about proper nutrition in other areas of your diet. Think about your lusts for a particular food, and think of them as being "crisis demands" by your system. But observe your cravings and what happens when you fulfill them—do you feel better over the long run, or worse? Remember that not all cravings are symptomatic of nutrient deficiencies. Often, food allergies or addictions can be the cause. In Chinese medicine, cravings are considered to be promoted by bodily imbalances.

Protein preferences

Red meat is sometimes a relatively easy craving to decode. Many women experience cravings for it around the time when they menstruate. Blood loss means reduced iron levels, and meat cravings can mean that your body's trying to prevent anemia. They can also mean that your body is building or repairing tissue.

If you're a meat eater, now is the time to indulge in a good-quality steak or even liver or other organ meats. If you're a vegetarian and you experience a craving for meat, overcome the chagrin of wanting something that you don't really wish to have by increasing your intake of plant-source protein, vitamin B_{12}, and iron.

If you're experiencing PMS symptoms as part of perimenopause or menopause, you can take a tip from women who have found that specific foods reduce their symptoms. Some women experience less menstrual pain when they increase their intake of animal and fish products, as well as their omega-3 fatty-acid intake. Other women find that easing off on coffee and other caffeine sources cuts their PMS problems and hot flashes as well. Still other women find relief from premenstrual bloat by eating low-fat diets. The flip side of that coin, however, is the fact that a low-fat diet generally means a diet higher in carbohydrates than it otherwise would be.

As a testament to the individuality of our systems, high carbohydrate intake correlates with irritability and other unfavorable emotional symptoms in some women who suffer PMS, but other women report decreased symptoms after they eat carbohydrates. It is likely that some women are more sensitive to the effects of carbohydrates than others. Perhaps a diet that is moderate in carbohydrate intake would better stabilize the situation.

The vegetarian view

Whether you are vegetarian for a specific reason or just tend to choose nonmeat foods by default, you should know a few things about how vegetarianism relates to your general health and also to menopause.

Ensuring adequate nutrition

Lacto-ovo-vegetarians, who include eggs and dairy products in their diets, may enjoy excellent health relatively effortlessly as long as they get adequate protein. *Vegans,* who eschew dairy products and eggs (essentially, anything from an animal source) may

Bright Idea
Anyone can use a little body wisdom. If a craving subsides when you feed yourself a substitute food (say, an essential-fatty-acid supplement and a mineral capsule when you're thinking chocolate), you've likely addressed the need that your body was trying to fill. Make a note of the result, and add appropriate preventative reinforcements to your diet.

Timesaver
Omega-3 fish-oil supplements are available in capsules at your local health-food store. Strict vegetarians may want to try flax oil, evening primrose oil, or other plant-based oils that are rich sources of essential fatty acids.

have greater challenges in meeting established dietary guidelines.

Planned food-combining to ensure adequate protein intake is a must. Because meat, fish, and poultry are major providers of iron, zinc, and B vitamins, vegetarians need to ensure that they get adequate quantities of these nutrients as well. Vitamin B_{12} is typically of animal origin, so outside supplementation is a necessity for vegans. Vitamin D and calcium levels should also be monitored. Fortunately, D is abundant in certain greens, such as arugula.

The dairy dilemma

Many people have difficulty digesting dairy products. In fact, some gynecologists link the use of dairy products to benign breast problems, vaginal discharge, acne, menstrual cramps, fibroids, chronic intestinal upset, and increased pain from endometriosis. So says Dr. Christine Northrup in her book *Women's Bodies, Women's Wisdom* (Bantam Books, 1994).

Yet many Americans get their daily calcium intake largely from dairy products, and for the health of their bones, milk and other dairy products *are* recommended foods. Studies suggest that increased dairy-calcium intake in premenopausal women may prevent age-related bone loss. Other studies, however, have found reduced rates of osteoporosis in vegetarians, suggesting that the need for calcium supplementation may be reduced among those who don't eat meat.

Are we getting enough?

When you're dealing with difficult symptoms during perimenopause and menopause, improving your

Watch Out!
Stress can increase your body's demand for a wide range of nutrients. Don't skimp on wholesome foods or supplements when stress prevails or during illness.

nutrition is a primary way to rule out *causes* of various problems. Many conditions can stem from deficiencies of various nutrients. Simply making sure that you're getting adequate amounts across the board can screen out these easily corrected situations. Even if your problems don't arise from deficiencies, adequate nutrition can only help your body repair damage.

Meeting all our nutrient needs by diet alone can be very difficult. Increased levels of stress and pollution, and reduced availability of some nutrients in the soil in which our food is grown, contribute to the dilemma. But along with a good multiple-vitamin-and-mineral supplement, simply being conscious of what you're eating can help. Start reading labels, and whenever possible, choose whole natural foods over highly processed ones.

Rather than simply keeping us from experiencing hunger, the meals that we eat sustain our bodies and capabilities. Thinking about what we put into our mouths is actually a large step toward health, and a simple one.

Just the facts

- Vitamin E may help ease hot flashes.

- Bone strength depends on many nutrients including calcium, vitamins A and D, copper, zinc, magnesium, manganese, and fluoride, to name a few.

- Diet and nutritional supplements may play a major role in preventing cancer, heart disease, and aging.

- Various amino acids, which are the building blocks of protein, are mood foods, countering nervousness and depression.

- Essential fatty acids are important in mood regulation.
- Adequate protein and a source of complex carbohydrates early in the day can often prevent mood dips in the afternoon and evening.

GET THE SCOOP ON...

Realistic lifestyle changes to help menopause ▪
Scientific reasons why happiness matters ▪
What kinds of exercise help and which don't ▪
Whether stress hastens menopause

Treating Menopause with Lifestyle

It seems obvious that when you're feeling at your best emotionally, and you're not steeped in worry or other negative emotions, your body can perform more closely to its optimal potential. What has become known as *mind-body medicine* has a firm grounding in common sense. Who decided that there should be a distinction between mind and body in the first place? Of *course* they affect each other, as scientists are discovering anew.

Stress reduction and adequate exercise are important in general good health and in many conditions, but they have a specific link to menopause. The basis of menopause is hormonal, and as you may recall, the substances that are so important in regulating a wide range of body activities are known as *stress* hormones.

This chapter explores the basics of a healthy relationship between your stress hormones and your sex hormones. The chapter also introduces a variety of mind-body approaches to help ease your

Chapter 11

menopausal passage—ranging from yoga and Tai Chi to simple aerobic exercise to specific stress-reduction techniques—and tells you *why* they do what they do in assisting your health.

The active, low-stress lifestyle

If anyone says, "You look so fresh, like you've just come back from vacation," think about it. When do you look and feel your best, and when are your appearance and comfort at their worst? Chances are that you'll find a correlation with stress somewhere in your life. A stress-free lifestyle doesn't allow you to fret about whether you're actually achieving it; part of the point is going with the flow.

We all thrive on stress, to some degree. Without a little of it, we would be inactive and lifeless. A tiny amount of stress can be a stimulus, drawing a response that engages body, mind, and spirit. With a little stress that we successfully handle, we grow. But coping with stress all day long, every day, is not good for anyone. By continually invoking our bodies' stress response mechanism—the *fight or flight response*—we're activating adrenaline and other hormones that are designed to be used in the human body mainly for emergencies. We also endanger the balance of our other hormones and the rest of our health in doing so.

Stress of the kind that's damaging to your health can take many forms. It doesn't take an extreme panic-inducing situation to hurt your health—just a chronic nag. Checklist 11.1 can help you summarize how much stress you really experience.

Despite what your mother may have told you about the virtue of being long suffering, no one benefits if you damage your body by trying to handle more than you really can. To be completely

Moneysaver
Many ways to counter stress (such as meditation) are free and good for you—unlike smoking, overeating, and other easy outs that may be tempting to try when you're feeling at the end of your wits.

CHECKLIST 11.1: WHAT ARE YOUR STRESSORS?

← Note!
Place a check beside all the stressors that you experience.

___ Stimulants (coffee and colas, for example)

___ Diet (unbalanced, caloric restriction, junk food, and so on)

___ Not enough sleep or insomnia

___ Busy schedule

___ Commuter annoyances

___ Relationship difficulties

___ Unpleasant physical surroundings

___ Illness

___ Medications

___ Excessive weight

___ Menopause-related stress (hormonal and menstrual irregularities and symptoms)

___ Other _____

healthy—physically, mentally, emotionally, and spiritually—you must be happy, comfortable, and thriving. Live by the tenet "Do unto others as you would have them do unto you," but make sure that you refrain from doing damage unto yourself, too!

Stress and premature menopause

It's well-known that smoking, chemotherapy, and other things that are hard on a woman's body can hasten menopause or exacerbate symptoms. But what about simple psychological stress? The intuitive answer is yes. A 1997 British study, conducted by the Department of Epidemiology and Public Health, surveyed more than 1,000 women and found that those who had the least education, those who had stressful lives, and those who had a history of poor physical and psychological health at age 36 reported more symptoms at age 47 than other women did.

Although stress can easily cause headaches, as we all know, there's now some evidence that it may shrivel the brain, too. A study published in the journal *Science* suggests that significant emotional upheavals may spur damaging changes in the hippocampus, which is the center of complex memory operations.

In addition, studies of patients who exhibit post-traumatic stress disorder, severe depression, and Cushing's syndrome all show high levels of glucocorticoid stress hormones. Brain scans reveal patterns of brain shrinkage when high levels of these hormones are present.

Stress is linked to accelerated aging in many ways, and inappropriate methods of countering stress can do us further harm—perhaps more than the stress itself would have. Excessive release of stress hormones can cause cardiovascular diseases and a host of other problems in older people. But according to a study done in Denmark under the auspices of the University of Copenhagen, the dysfunctional ways in which we try to cope with stress may cause more ill health than the body's own hypersecretion of the stress hormones epinephrine and cortisol. The study's authors, N. J. Christensen and E. W. Jensen, suggest that dysfunctional coping strategies are largely responsible for the harmful effects of stress. Although the study focused on smoking, which correlated with an increase in norepinephrine and other stress hormones, it's easy to come up with any number of dysfunctional coping strategies.

The restorative powers of stress reduction
Research is beginning to confirm what many people suspect: that lowering stress levels can truly

aid healing and prevent further disease. One recent study at Duke University, reported in the American Medical Association's *Archives of Internal Medicine*, showed that heart patients dramatically lowered their risk of further cardiac problems by using simple stress-reduction techniques.

In the Duke study, 107 heart patients were divided into three groups: a control group, which received normal heart care; a group that embarked on a four-month exercise program; and a group that took part in a four-month stress-reduction program. In the latter group, participants attended a 90-minute de-stressing lesson every week.

In the group that received normal physicians' care, 12 of the 40 patients experienced a cardiac event (heart attack or heart surgery). In the exercise group, 7 of 34 experienced a cardiac event. But only 3 of the 33 participants in the stress-reduction group suffered a cardiac event, which made them 74 percent less likely to have further heart difficulties than patients who received routine medical follow-up care.

The benefits of stress reduction stretch far beyond helping the heart. Just as how your hormone levels affect how you feel, how you feel can affect your hormone levels. Hormones are intimately tied up in how we deal with our day-to-day world, how we feel about our lives, and how we feel about ourselves, and there is no faking out our systems. Genuine happiness and comfort are necessities for health.

In *Women's Bodies Women's Wisdom*, Christiane Northrup, M.D., writes that negative feelings about being female, and feelings of being subordinate and inferior, actually cause some women to

Bright Idea
Develop one healthy stress-reduction technique that you can use for each major stressor that you experience every day. For noise pollution, consider music. For interpersonal difficulties, try affirmations or something else that enhances your self-esteem.

Watch Out!
Make sure that your nutritional needs are well met when you're under stress. Daily worries, illness, or anything that activates your stress response prompts your body to use inordinate quantities of vitamins and other nutrients, so less material is left over for normal repair and maintenance.

stop ovulating and become more androgynous. She notes that studies of female monkeys showed that those who were in a position of social subordination often underwent ovarian difficulties.

Indeed, in animal settings, social standing is interwoven with hormones. Social prominence in females correlates with high estrogen levels, and the same holds true for testosterone in males. And as social roles change, so does hormone status. A study of red-winged blackbirds, for example, finds that even variations in birdsong correlate with lower or higher sex-hormone levels, with higher levels leading to both increased aggression and sexual display in males.

De-stressing your life

The first step to managing stress in your life is realizing where it is. Think about the stressors in Checklist 11.1 that apply to you (refer to "The active, low-stress lifestyle" earlier in this chapter). Is it the disorganized environment you're in that subtly gets on your nerves all the time, or is it the horrendous commute through rush-hour traffic every day? Is your diet lacking solid nutrition? (If you feel a lack of energy by early afternoon, it may be.) Or do you have unresolved issues with another person?

When you figure out what's really bugging you, you can start taking steps to alleviate the pressure. Look at how you deal with stress. Do you employ good coping strategies or bad ones? Checklist 11.2 shows how your choices stack up.

Take a moment to write down specific stressors in your life and how you tend to cope with each one. Do you eat junk food after the difficult drive home from work, have a glass of beer to help you forget about a difficult co-worker, or spend too much

CHECKLIST 11.2: HOW DO YOU COPE WITH STRESS?

Negative Strategies	Positive Strategies
____ Indulging bitterness, anger, frustration, or other negative emotions	____ Reevaluating your priorities
____ Overeating	____ Engaging in relaxing activities (long baths, reading, or listening to music, for example)
____ Smoking or abusing other substances	____ Making dietary changes to include mood foods (refer to Chapter 10)
____ Drinking alcohol	____ Engaging in physical exercise
____ Dropping out (letting yourself collapse and withdraw emotionally)	____ Spending time with caring, supportive friends
____ Ignoring your normal day-to-day chores (skipping the housework, for example)	____ Making an effort to clean up or even enrich your immediate environment

← Note!
Shifting from a negative response to stress to one that is more positive not only reduces your current stress level, but also reduces your susceptibility to future stress reactions.

shopping when the dollars might have been better spent on a massage or a more comfortable chair for your home office?

Eliminate the negative

You may be able to eliminate some stressors, such as a particularly rough commute to work. You really can't eliminate some other stressors, such as your children. Make a list of your top-five minor day-to-day stressors in your life; then make a list of the top-five deep, serious stressors that you face—things more serious than annoyances, such as the illness of a loved one or ongoing difficulty in communicating with your spouse.

Starting with your list of daily annoyances, spend a few calm minutes jotting down notes about how to modify or eliminate the problem. Table 11.1 shows an example.

TABLE 11.1: REDUCING DAILY STRESS

Stressor	Ways to Modify It
Commuting	1. Take a more scenic, less crowded route home, even if the drive takes longer.
	2. Arrange to leave home earlier (and work later) to avoid rush-hour traffic.
	3. Consider finding work closer to home.
Hot flashes	1. Explore dietary and herbal-therapy changes.
	2. Talk to supportive people (friends, support groups, and even Internet chat groups) who understand what you're going through.
	3. Be prepared. Carry cooling towelettes in your purse, wear layered clothing so that you can shed a jacket or sweater when you need to, and install adequate air-conditioning or fans.
Too-busy schedule	1. Reprioritize, cutting or delegating tasks whenever possible.
	2. Learn to pace yourself. Find or make time for breaks, and take them anywhere *except* in your office or workplace.
	3. Build stress-busting elements into your routine. Play your favorite music in your office or on your car radio, or adjust your desk lighting to a comfortable level.

The more you can eliminate day-to-day stress, the less other stressors should affect you. You can often reduce daily stress just by making a few rearrangements. The serious stressors in your life are usually best dealt with when you've regained a measure of comfort and composure and can think clearly about what to do. For now, know that you're headed in the right direction.

To sleep, perchance to dream

The average amount of sleep that adults get every night is believed to be hours less now than hundreds of years ago. But how much is enough? Eight hours? Six hours? The only number that really matters is how much sleep *you* thrive on.

Sleep is one area in which you should trust your body's wisdom. Some people need 6 hours every night; others need as many as 12. The necessary amount of sleep varies from person to person. Some people are natural early risers, whereas others wouldn't be caught dead getting up early if they didn't have to. Infants (who sleep about 18 hours every day) and people who are recovering from illness typically require significantly more sleep than do normal, healthy adults, who average about 7 hours of nightly sleep.

The *kind* of sleep that you get matters as well. Infants, for example, have a high proportion of REM sleep (the deep sleep in which dreams occur) to light sleep. They're actually in REM sleep about half the time when they're not awake! Compare that statistic with the typical adult REM session of just 2 hours. To get your rest, you need REM sleep, which means having a solid night of being knocked out to reach deep levels, rather than occasionally waking or just taking naps that equal several hours of sleep.

Insomnia is a frequent annoyance during perimenopause and menopause. Insomnia is often the result of hot flashes that occur during sleep. You may find yourself suddenly awakened from a sound sleep with perspiration on your brow and an intense desire to throw off the covers. Sometimes these hot flashes occur several times each night. The resulting sleep deprivation leads to irritability, inability to concentrate, and a general feeling of malaise.

Bright Idea
Add a form of meditation to your daily routine, and use it as a quick break from stressful situations or when you have trouble concentrating. According to the Vivekananda Kendra Yoga Research Foundation in Bangalore, India, focused meditation can simultaneously increase mental alertness and reduce the heart rate.

Tackling this frustrating symptom should be high on your list of ways to de-stress your life and improve your passage. Sometimes behavior modification can improve this kind of insomnia, though sometimes readjustment of hormone levels is needed.

Watch Out!
If your insomnia is persistent and serious, discuss it with your doctor. Without adequate sleep, you can't expect to function well during the day— or all the way through menopause. On the Web, you can discuss sleep problems in the newsgroup alt.support. sleep-disorder.

Sleep helps stabilize brain activity. Studies of the Arctic ground squirrel suggest that each hour of sleep stabilizes brain synapses for as long as four hours. The different states of sleep are controlled by your thalamus, hypothalamus, brain, and basal forebrain, and your patterns of waking and falling asleep are largely controlled by the thalamus. Your hormones are also at work and play as an integral part of the sleep-wake cycle.

Your level of wakefulness is determined by the following:

- Acetylcholine

- Serotonin

- Histamine

- Norepinephrine

Prolactin, which is a key hormone in the production of breast milk (*prolactin* means *pro-lactation*), may help stimulate deep REM sleep. Growth-hormone-releasing hormone affects other phases of sleep, and serotonin receptors are important during light sleep.

You should be careful with anything that you take to induce sleep, and check with your doctor about more than occasional use. Alcohol is not a good option, not only because of its health risks, but also because it can actually reduce the amount of deep REM sleep that you get. A better idea is to get your own natural daily rhythms in sync. After you establish a good base, your out-of-sync menopausal hormones may be better able to follow along.

GETTING A GOOD NIGHT'S SLEEP

Set a regular bedtime—*before* midnight.

Try to wake up at the same time each day.

Avoid caffeine and other stimulants late in the day (or entirely).

Avoid excessive light in the evening and insufficient light during the daytime.

Review your medications and health supplements with your physician, and adjust the ones that may adversely affect your ability to sleep.

Avoid alcohol and other depressants.

Include exercise, and perhaps meditation, in your daily routine.

Exercise early in the day, using your evening hours for more-relaxing pursuits.

Keep your evening meal light, and avoid eating just before bedtime.

Make your bedroom a cozy place that encourages sleep. Soothing colors, good ventilation, and fluffy pillows all help.

Look into herbal and other folk remedies that promote relaxation and sleepiness (see Chapter 13).

Consider taking melatonin tablets as a sleep aid.

Timesaver
Need to adjust the times when you naturally fall asleep and awaken? Melatonin can reset your 24-hour circadian clock, turning it forward a little when taken at dusk or back a little when taken at dawn. For this reason, melatonin is useful for treating jet lag.

Take care of yourself

Beyond getting enough sleep, you have many common-sense ways to eliminate unnecessary stress from your life. If you smoke, stop; find a program that helps you quit definitively. Include healthy foods in your diet. (Check out Chapter 10 to learn about balancing your intake of nutrients, avoiding insulin surges and the resulting fatigue, and eating specific foods to support your moods.) Go easy on caffeine, too. And stop expecting to be Superwoman. You need only be one healthy, happy woman, whoever she happens to be.

Watch Out!
Neither mela-
tonin nor herbs
are without their
potential draw-
backs. For
instance, some
physicians warn
that takig mela-
tonin could exac-
erbate seasonal
depression. And
a small percent-
age of people
taking melatonin
have reported
nightmares,
headaches,
sleepiness in the
morning and
even lowered
libido. Remember
it is a hormone.

In short, take time to take care of yourself, and respect yourself exactly as you are. You can find pleasure in little things, so don't be afraid to indulge yourself. Make sure that your home is your castle, a comfortable retreat in which at least one room is your domain, filled with things that you love and where you love to be. Don't always schedule a roster of activities that have to be completed on Saturdays or Sundays; head off and explore, or just putter. Get as much real beauty into your life as you can.

Although job and career stress can exact a heavy toll on the female system (not to mention the male system), remember that if you are a wage earner, you also may be less affected by the stresses that earlier generations of women faced, such as having to rely on someone else for income or lack of intellectual fulfillment. (Not all women had those problems, of course.)

As you approach the concerns in your daily life, at work or at home, remember not to fit into some-one else's mold. If your gut tells you to take a caring approach on a business issue, rather than lock horns (and stimulate stress-hormone response), use both your mind *and* your emotions to handle things in the way that you see fit. If you experience less stress by taking a direct approach rather than continually trying to work things out, as many women do, act on your convictions. Your life is about you, not about behaving otherwise. Being true to yourself counters stress.

Exercise and meditation

Two of the best ways to help your body and mind adapt to stress are exercise and meditation, both of which can be conscious forms of relaxation. Are they work? Yes. But they pay off in pleasure and health.

Getting regular physical activity greatly reduces the risk of dying from coronary heart disease, the leading cause of death in the United States. It also cuts your chances of developing diabetes, hypertension, and colon cancer. Exercise enhances mental health; fosters healthy muscles, bones, and joints; and helps maintain body functions and preserve independence in old age.

According to the U.S. Surgeon General, Americans aren't getting enough exercise. Among the major conclusions of a report on physical activity are the following

■ People of all ages, both male and female, benefit from regular physical activity.

■ More than 60 percent of American adults are not regularly physically active. In fact, 25 percent of all adults are not active at all.

■ You can gain significant health benefits by including a moderate amount of physical activity on most, if not all, days of the week. Examples of moderate activity are 30 minutes of brisk walking or raking leaves, 15 minutes of running, or 45 minutes of playing volleyball. By modestly increasing your daily activity, you can improve your health and your quality of life.

■ You get additional health benefits from increasing your level of physical activity—upping the intensity or increasing the duration of your normal regimen.

■ Regular physical activity reduces the risk of premature mortality in general and of coronary heart disease, hypertension, colon cancer, and diabetes mellitus in particular. It also improves mental health and is important for the health of muscles, bones, and joints.

Bright Idea
Stop expecting the world of yourself, and start noticing the amazing things *in* your world. Your body and your emotions will respond with thanks.

One of the first steps that you can take to protect your health during menopause and beyond is to make certain that you're not among the one in four adults who are sedentary. Build activity into your day, either by starting a formal fitness program that is appropriate for your level of ability or at least by moving more. Fifteen minutes of activity twice (or even once) a day will help if you're consistent about it. Consider the following activities:

- Taking a short walk during your lunch break
- Doing a little gardening
- Performing simple exercises while you're watching the news
- Planning weekend outings that involve walking, bicycling, or other active sightseeing
- Washing your car and detailing the interior

Even embarking on the cleaning projects that you've been putting off can help get you into better shape. The more engaging the activity is, the less you'll notice that you're actually exercising. In the interest of ensuring a truly comfortable and stress-free environment at home, consider embarking on a renovation project. Go shopping for new linens, sort out the closet, rearrange the furniture, and so on. Make yourself a haven, and get some activity benefits in the process. In short, do things that you really want to do and gain fruitful results from. Don't discount the mind-body benefit of being fully engaged in something fun.

Effects on your hormones

Aerobic activity, such as running, can create a pleasure response in your body by releasing endorphins, and of course, it has other positive effects too. A comparison of running and meditation found both to be mood-elevating activities that stimulate the release of cortisol, a hormone that helps with adaptation during stress.

Many forms of exercise and simple mindful meditation help a variety of psychological conditions. A little attention to this area of your life can pay off in reducing stress and ameliorating the anxiety, depression, and mood instabilities that accompany menopause for many women.

One psychiatric study found that most patients experienced relief of anxiety and depression following a two-month stress-reduction program based on mindfulness meditation. Further study by researchers affiliated with the University of Massachusetts Medical Center found that the improvements were maintained even three years later.

The benefits of exercise

Including several kinds of exercise in your routine is beneficial. Aerobic activity (such as cycling and walking) benefits your cardiovascular system. Stretching keeps your muscles limber. Weight-bearing exercise (walking qualifies in this category, too) helps your future bone health, and a little weight lifting or some floor exercises tone your muscles.

One important factor in choosing an exercise program is how much you enjoy it. Taking a long walk at sunset every couple of days may do you more good in the long run than trying to go to a noisy gym where you don't like being. If you try yoga or dance, you may find that these activities do a fantastic job of building lean muscle, and they may be more appealing to you than working weight machines.

Your level of physical ability is another important factor to consider. If you're sturdy and in fine

Unofficially...
Although cortisol levels rise during stress, they help regulate energy balance. Elevated cortisol during exercise is considered to be appropriate, as long as cortisol isn't continually elevated.

Unofficially...
For many people, exercising becomes a form of meditation. Other people benefit from specific types of meditation that don't involve much physical exertion.

health, all the possibilities are open to you. If your range of mobility is limited, or if you must take it easier for another reason, water aerobics may be a good option. You may also want to try long walks, stretching, or the low-exertion but high-results Tai Chi.

With your doctor's approval, experiment with various activities. Try a yoga class, pick up a book on Tai Chi, or arrange some outings that require you to move more. Table 11.2 lists some exercise and meditation options. Note that some forms of yoga and other types of training may produce cardiovascular and aerobic benefits, but only exercises that are primarily aerobic in nature are noted as such in Table 11.2. Although many forms of exercise can produce meditation benefits, only those that are specifically geared to meditation are so marked in the table.

If you get bored doing things by yourself, persuade a friend to join you on a regular basis, or take a class rather than doing things on your own. If finances permit, consider exercising with a personal trainer. The right trainer will motivate you to achieve your goals, show you the proper way to exercise (especially important in preventing injury), and hopefully keep you on track. The commitment that accompanies working with a trainer may be the jump start you need.

After you try different forms of exercise and meditation, see where you notice benefits, and trust your body's intuition. Remember that there are many forms of exercise and meditation, beyond those described in this section. Go exploring!

The importance of weight-bearing exercise

Exercise in which you gently rely on your bones encourages them to maintain solidity, which can

TABLE 11.2: EXERCISE AND MEDITATION METHODS

Exercise	Aerobic	Muscle-Toning	Weight-Bearing	Meditation Benefits	Notes
Running	X	X	X	N/A	N/A
Walking	X	X	X	N/A	N/A
Aerobics classes	X	X	X	N/A	N/A
Cycling	X	X	N/A	N/A	N/A
Water aerobics	X	X	N/A	N/A	Excellent for people who have limited mobility or arthritis (check with your local YMCA or hospital wellness center for class locations)
Weight lifting	N/A	X	X	N/A	N/A
Yoga	N/A	X	N/A	X	Excellent for stress reduction and balance
Tai Chi	N/A	X	N/A	X	Excellent for stress reduction and balance; especially good for people who have arthritis or limited mobility
Qi Gong	N/A	X	N/A	X	Excellent for stress reduction

help reduce your risk of osteoporosis. The motto in this regard is "Use it or lose it." Anyone who is experiencing thinning bones should be particularly careful about high-impact exercise (as we all should, frankly).

Because putting weight on your leg bones isn't likely to help your arm bones, getting a variety of weight-bearing exercise is ideal. Weight lifting is, of course, weight-bearing exercise, but calisthenics and many aerobic activities qualify as well. Are you putting some weight on your bones when you perform an activity? If so, the activity is weight-bearing exercise.

Weight-bearing exercise not only tends to stimulate the formation of new bone, but also strengthens the muscles that support your bones, making you less likely to break a bone. (It also improves your balance.) As always, be prudent, and seek your physician's advice about safe exercise for your present level of bone health.

Watch Out!
Don't overdo weight-bearing exercise. Putting too much stress on your bones can break them down instead of build them up.

Antistress offerings from the East

American culture has been both lauded and criticized for its emphasis on productivity and activity. In terms of the Asian concepts of yin and yang, you can view Western ways as being quite yang, without much concentration on restorative, conservative yin.

It's no surprise, then, that many of the most popular stress-reduction techniques originated in Asia, where a holistic view has been around literally for ages. This section explains some seemingly mysterious techniques from the Orient.

Yoga for menopause

If you don't know much about yoga, you may think of it as being just another form of exercise—perhaps a gentle one that's good for stretching your muscles and toning up, but not much more. Yoga, however, originated thousands of years ago in India as an exercise in spirituality. Yogis, who were the first practitioners of yoga, took their exercises religiously. In fact, the Sanskrit word *yoga* means *union*.

At the most basic physical level, yoga is about breathing and focus. Steady, rhythmic deep breathing sees you through increasingly arduous stances. If you concentrate on relaxing and inhaling deeply, yoga gets easier. Many people say that they leave their classes feeling calm or even euphoric

Practicing yoga regularly is suggested to have a beneficial effect on hormone balance. One study reviewed the experiences of participants in a three-month residential yoga and meditation program. The participants took yoga classes, meditated, and ate a low-fat semivegetarian diet. By the end of the study, the researchers found substantial reduction in risk factors. The participants' cardiovascular results improved, as did their ratios of lean to fat tissue. Cholesterol levels and blood pressure also dropped. In addition the researchers found decreased levels of stress hormone production suggesting that the participants either experienced less stress or managed it better.

Doing yoga may help with your other activities and forms of exercise as well, particularly by making your cardiorespiratory efforts more efficient. In a study conducted by the Vemana Yoga Research Institute of Hyderabad, India, six healthy adult women did four weeks of intensive yoga practice (two 90-minute sessions a day) and then were tested on a treadmill. Maximal work output increased by 21 percent, and the level of oxygen consumption in

Unofficially...
There are many kinds of yoga, and they use a variety of movement styles. Yoga usually is practiced on a thin foam mat, and participants wear comfortable, loose clothing to allow unrestricted movement.

Bright Idea
Before you
decide on a sin-
gle type of yoga,
look for a yoga
center where you
feel that you'd
be comfortable
taking classes.
Also try your
local YMCA and
area gyms, and
get advice from
teachers and
other students.

relation to output decreased significantly. The test subjects were able to do more exercise than before, without raising their heart rates considerably.

Tai Chi: Slow moves for great benefits

Tai Chi is an age-old Asian meditation and fitness technique that is ideal for reducing stress and developing balance. Tai Chi is also called *T'ai Chi Ch'uan* or *Taijiquan*, which translates loosely as "Supreme Ultimate." It involves concentration and flow, and when practiced correctly, it produces benefits without overexertion.

In Asia, Tai Chi breaks and miniclasses are often held in workplaces. In the United States, you may find Tai Chi classes at your local YMCA, hospital wellness centers, martial-arts schools, and even senior-citizens' organizations, as well as at centers that offer yoga classes.

You can use Tai Chi to help lower high blood pressure. Certain stances (such as the low bent-knee position) have been shown to stimulate the cardiovascular system without straining joints, muscles, or connective tissues.

Qi Gong

Qi Gong is another ancient Eastern form of meditation and exercise, believed to have its roots in China at least a dozen centuries before Christ. Qi Gong was practiced by early Chinese Taoists as well as by Indian Buddhists, and it remains popular in modern Asian countries today (as well as elsewhere in the world).

Qi Gong (also called *Chi Kung*) means c*ultivating the life force* or w*orking the energy*. The practice involves deep breathing and exercises that are designed to circulate energy (known as *Qi* and pronounced "chee") throughout the body. The moves produce intentional tension, followed by relaxation. Visualization techniques are also used. About 150 forms of Qi Gong exist.

Although Western medicine hasn't confirmed the existence of *Qi* or of the bodily channels through which Asian health philosophy says it travels, give *Qi*-related exercises a try. Keep an open mind. If you see results, you see results.

To do Qi Gong and other exercises and forms of meditation properly, take a formal class. Learning the basics from a qualified instructor can ensure that you're practicing it properly. Then you can go on your own, if you want.

You can sample a bit of Qi Gong–based exercise on your own, however, by gently performing the following moves:

1. Take a deep breath, and stand with your feet about shoulder width apart, knees bent a little.

2. Take another slow, deep breath, and then let your breath out slowly while you reach upward with one arm, flexing your hand.

3. Holding the pose, inhale slowly.

4. After about 10 seconds, exhale, and at the same time, lower your arm and raise the other one.

5. Repeat the preceding steps, alternating arms.

You can also try this Qi Gong exercise:

1. Standing with your feet about shoulder width apart, bend your knees a little, and let your upper body hang downward comfortably.

2. Relaxing your back and using your leg muscles, slowly roll your upper body back toward a standing position while inhaling.

Timesaver
For a short course on the workings of *Qi* (not to mention *Jing* and *Shen*), see Chapter 13 for a discussion of herbs and Chinese medicine.

3. At about hip level, cross your arms (touching each elbow with the other hand), and keep rising.

4. At about shoulder level, uncross your arms, and extend them upward and outward in a joyful stretch as you reach and exhale.

5. Repeat the preceding steps a few times.

Another form of Qi Gong is described in Chapter 13. Like massage, this form of Qi Gong involves a therapist; it's not a program that you perform yourself.

Breath work

A specific exercise done in yoga and Qi Gong, *alternate breathing*, has yielded interesting results with regard to improvement in mental function. Yoga experts believe that rhythmic inhalation, first through one nostril and then through the other, affects right-brain and left-brain function. Studies have shown that this technique can be useful for certain psychiatric conditions (such as obsessive-compulsive disorder), reducing patients' reliance on medication.

In another study, conducted by the Vivekananda Kendra Yoga Research Foundation, students practiced right-nostril breathing, left-nostril breathing, alternate-nostril breathing, or breath awareness without concentration on a particular nostril. After 10 days, the students asked to take tests evaluating their verbal and spatial memory. A control group that did take part in the breathing exercises took the same tests. All four of the groups that performed breathing exercises showed significant increases in their spatial test scores—an average 84 percent increase, in comparison with no increase in score for the control group. The study concluded that yoga breathing may increase spatial rather than verbal scores, suggesting it enhances activity in the part of the brain responsible for processing visual information. That is, it appears to enhance activity in the part of the brain responsible for processing visual information like depth perception.

In 1997, a team of German researchers tested the bodily equilibrium of study participants who were watching disorienting optical patterns on a video screen. The subjects were asked to shift their postures at different intervals. The participants who had engaged in breath work showed significantly better coordination than did members of the control group, who had done no breath work. The study suggests that breath work is a valuable method for treatment and rehabilitation of balance disorders.

More conventional forms of yoga can also greatly assist with developing balance, both physical and spiritual, in the body. And balancing your body and emotions—as yoga and other meditative forms of exercise have been found to do—can lead to balancing your hormones by reducing stress and increasing a sense of well-being.

The mind–body connection

Mainstream medicine is beginning to embrace a more holistic outlook. Although plenty of controversy still exists, scientific studies and clinical results are making headway in convincing skeptics of the interplay of our thoughts, emotions, and physical health.

What we think and how we feel directly affect the release and use of neurotransmitters, hormones, and other body messengers. Our mental and emotional processes do not happen

> **❝**
> It would be possible to describe everything scientifically, but it would make no sense; it would be without meaning, as if you described a Beethoven symphony as a variation of wave pressure.
> —Albert Einstein
> **❞**

independently of chemistry; instead, they rely on it and even change it.

The idea that we can activate a "vast internal pharmacy" through our thoughts, feelings, and actions is underscored by medical knowledge of basic physiology.

Further reaches of mind-body medicine, however, are not so widely accepted. One disputed concept is whether prayer or good wishes from someone else can directly improve health. Science does not yet know why this happens, if and when it does. Several studies (criticized, however, for their methods) have addressed the impact of prayer on real physical healing.

Spiritually speaking

A famous study by cardiologist Randolph C. Byrd, M.D., conducted during the early 1980s, tested the intercessory power of outside daily prayer groups in the recovery of nearly 400 heart-attack patients. In "Positive Therapeutic Effects of Intercessory Prayer in a Coronary Care Unit Population," Byrd reported that fewer patients in the group that was prayed for required ventilatory support, antibiotics, or diuretics. A complicated hospital course of treatment was observed in 14 percent of the prayer group as compared to 22 percent of the control group. Based on the data, Byrd concluded that intercessional prayer seemed to have a beneficial effect.

Among the criticisms of the study, however, was that there was no way of knowing whether relatives or family members actually prayed for the control group. Other studies on prayer showed negative, neutral, or positive results, and so the topic remains slippery and undecided as far as science is concerned.

There's room for benefit from a positive attitude, however, whether your belief in mind-body medicine is limited to the provable fact that your mind influences the matter portion of your body, or whether your spirituality supports the concept of prayer and other practices as being beneficial.

Charting the mind-body response

The concept of *biofeedback* was introduced during the 1960s, when experimental psychologists demonstrated that people could learn to change some body processes.

Biofeedback techniques are still used today to treat a variety of problems, including the following:

- Addictions

- Anxiety

- Asthma

- Headaches (including migraines)

- Heart problems

- High blood pressure

- Hot flashes

- Incontinence

- Indigestion and irritable-bowel syndrome

- Insomnia

- Menstrual irregularities

In the case of menstrual irregularities (dysmenorrhea), biofeedback-assisted relaxation has been reported to alleviate pain and discomfort in conditions that resisted treatment with either hormones or painkillers.

At its simplest, biofeedback lets you know when you're meditating and relaxing properly, so that your body can access its own pharmaceuticals that make you feel better and assist healing.

> **"**
> The arrival of a good clown exercises a more beneficial influence upon the health of a town than the arrival of twenty asses laden with drugs.
> —17th-century physician Thomas Sydenham
> **"**

Biofeedback in a clinical setting often involves the use of monitoring devices to check the following items:

- Skin temperature
- Muscle tension
- Respiration patterns and rate
- Brain-wave patterns

To get the effect of the helpful alpha brain-wave pattern at home, gear your meditation and relaxation to doing less conscious thinking about the activities of the day. Deeper meditative contemplation tends to evoke the also-helpful theta brain-wave state. Both states should do you more good in meditative efforts than the busy beta state, in which we conduct much of our lives.

Chapter 13 describes more mind-body therapies that you can use for healthy hormones during menopause.

Just the facts

- Stress is linked with accelerated aging and increased menopausal problems.

- Meditation and aerobic exercise have been found to have some of the same benefits, and both practices may help stabilize hormone levels.

- Weight-bearing exercise improves the solidity of your bones and helps prevent osteoporosis.

- The production and use of stress hormones is intimately tied to the production and use of sex hormones in our bodies.

GET THE SCOOP ON...

Prescription drugs for hot flashes ▪ Over-the-counter remedies for typical menopausal symptoms ▪ Osteoporosis protection without hormones ▪ Why you may choose to treat just your symptoms ▪ Hysterectomy—a last resort?

Nonhormone Treatment from Conventional Medicine

W hether you're taking hormone-replacement therapy (HRT) or choose not to, you should be aware of other conventional medical treatments for problems that often occur during perimenopause and menopause. Rather than address the underlying issue of hormones, your physician can prescribe medications to treat your symptoms, ranging from hot flashes to insomnia. He or she can also prescribe other medications to help prevent osteoporosis and curb other conditions for which postmenopausal women are at risk.

There are many reasons women may choose to treat menopause symptoms with medications other than HRT. Some women, particularly those whose difficulties are not severe, may prefer to treat only their symptoms. Sometimes anxiety about potential risks prevents women from using HRT. Other women may want to take HRT but may not be candidates for it due to preexisting medical conditions. Also, some women using HRT discover a perfect fit with hormones and dosages can be hard to find, and thus they may need additional support for their symptoms.

In other words, despite that extra estrogen, a hot flash is still a hot flash, and when you get one, you want relief. This chapter outlines some major conventional ways that you can treat typical menopause difficulties without HRT.

Hot flashes and headaches

Hot flashes are easily the symptom that is most frequently associated with menopause. They are the body's reaction to decreased levels of estrogen and are perceived as a sudden rush of intense warmth in the upper body. Hot flashes generally last for several minutes (usually 2–4 minutes duration). There is variation amongst women in the number of hot flashes per day, the intensity of symptoms, and the duration in years that hot flashes persist. Flashes are generally more intense if there is a sudden and dramatic decrease in estrogen levels, as occurs in a surgical menopause (that is, after surgical removal of the ovaries). Hot flashes frequently begin during the late perimenopausal years, when estrogen levels begin to decrease. Hot flashes can persist for 5–10 years after the last period, although most women experience them for less than 5 years, with 1–2 years being the most common. Hot flashes can be triggered by emotional situations such as stress or anxiety.

Hot flashes typically involve increased heart rate, elevated temperature, and a flush of more than usual blood flow through the upper body.

Therefore, medications that bring down fevers, lower high blood pressure, and stabilize heart rate can often be used as treatment.

While hormones are the only FDA-approved medications for treatment of hot flashes, physicians have the option of prescribing other medications to treat these symptoms. These medications do not have the same proven track record for relieving hot flashes when compared to estrogen, but they may prove beneficial to you as long as they don't interact with other medications or cause any adverse side effects. You can discuss several options with your doctor, including medications such as the following:

- Antihypertensives, which lower blood pressure)

- Antidepressants and antianxiety agents

- Bellergal-S (a combination of medicines)

Your physician may suggest or even prescribe vitamin E for hot flashes. See the chapters on nutrition (Chapter 10) and herbs (Chapter 13) for more information about vitamins and alternative treatments.

Sometimes, hot flashes can be accompanied by headaches. Migraine headaches, which affect about 25 million people in the United States each year, have been linked in women to changing estrogen levels. Prior to menopause they are frequently seen during times of hormone fluctuation, such as the days preceding a menstrual period. In a similar fashion, during menopause, the hormonal fluctuations associated with hot flashes can sometimes trigger a migraine headache.

Some treatments that are effective for controlling other hot-flash symptoms can help with the headache part. Look for a therapy that specifically offers *analgesic* (painkilling) properties, or consider

Unofficially...
The more body fat you have, the less likely you are to have hot flashes (technically speaking) because the body can use the estrogen that is formed in fat when other reserves are running low. Obese women tend to have less severe hot flashes than their thinner counterparts do.

adding an over-the-counter analgesic to what you take for a hot flash. But check with your doctor or pharmacist first to make sure that the medications are compatible.

Blood-pressure medications

Physicians sometimes prescribe antihypertensives (medications that lower blood pressure) to help reduce the severity of hot flashes. Because hypertension is high blood pressure, these drugs may best be used if you tend to experience elevated blood pressure anyway. If, however, your blood pressure runs low to begin with, antihypertensives may not be the best approach.

Antihypertensive medications have been used to treat hot flashes. The medical term for hot flashes is "vasomotor instability" which literally means unstable blood vessel reactions. Antihypertensive medicines help to stabilize the blood vessels and often decrease rapid heart rates associated with hot flashes. By far, the most effective agent is Clonidine (Catapres), which is best administered as a transdermal patch (100 micrograms applied once each week). It has been shown to be more effective than placebo (sugar pills) in several studies. Side effects include mouth dryness, constipation, and skin irritation from the patch.

Discuss with your doctor if this medication is safe for you to use.

Other hot-flash treatments

A drug known as Bellergal-S is approved by the U.S. Food and Drug Administration for treating hot flashes. This drug—which consists of belladonna, ergotamine, and phenobarbital—typically is appropriate only for short-term use because phenobarbital (a barbiturate) can be addictive. Bellergal-S is

Timesaver
Adults are considered to have hypertension when their blood pressure is at least 140 mm Hg systolic and at least 90 mm Hg diastolic, according to the American Heart Association. Most people are familiar with this reading as "140/90" or "140 over 90."

available only as a generic medication and is no longer listed in the Physicians Desk Reference (PDR). The dosage is one tablet in the morning and one tablet in the evening. Its benefit is limited to *short term* management of hot flashes, restlessness, anxiety, sweating, and insomnia. It will also help prevent migraine headaches.

Women with breast cancer who experience hot flashes are usually not candidates for HRT. The topic of HRT for these women is controversial, but for now most physicians are reluctant to prescribe it. For those women experiencing debilitating hot flashes treatment with megace (megestrol acetate), a type of progestin, will generally result in improvement. Side effects include occasional chills and weight gain. Experience with this medicine in women without breast cancer is limited and is not reccomended at this time.

Studies show significant benefit from relaxation in treating menopausal hot flashes. Groups trained in relaxation techniques had less intense and less frequent hot flashes as well as reductions in anxiety and depression.

Over-the-counter options

When hot flashes are bad enough to make you reach for the medicine cabinet, what over-the-counter treatments should you look for? Generally, you can find some relief from the same things that you may have taken to relieve premenstrual discomfort, including the following:

- Aspirin
- Ibuprofen
- Ketoprofen
- Naproxen sodium

Unofficially... The plant belladonna is highly poisonous, but the belladonna alkaloids used in Bellergal-S are safely used in other medications, and are paired with barbiturates to relieve stomach and intestinal cramping.

Bright Idea
To counter hot flashes, you can try relaxation strategies, making the room cooler, and dressing in layers so that you can peel off clothing as needed. Also watch your intake of spicy foods, alcohol, and caffeine since these substances can trigger hot flashes.

All four remedies can be effective in relieving headaches and fever. Acetaminophen can help as well, and is less likely to cause stomach problems. These products, known collectively as nonsteroidal anti-inflammatory drugs (*NSAIDs*), are sold under many brand names, and they comprise a huge portion of the over-the-counter analgesics that are available. All of them *do* have side effects, including gastric irritation and possible kidney damage. For this reason, they should be used intermittently, not chronically.

Check labels, and consider products that are not paired with caffeine when you're using them. (Look for the brand that offers the most convenient dosing schedule, too.) Although caffeine can enhance the effectiveness of painkillers, it has also been found to trigger or worsen some hot-flash and migraine symptoms. Everyone's hot flashes are different. It may be worthwhile to try a caffeine-added brand one time and a caffeine-free preparation another time to see which brings you the most relief.

Aspirin is believed to work by inhibiting the release of prostaglandins, which regulate blood-vessel elasticity and some functions of blood platelets. Consequently, it can reduce inflammation and inhibit blood clotting.

Musings on migraines

Migraine headaches are thought in some cases to be related to fluctuating estrogen levels. But other things can trigger or exacerbate migraines—something to keep in mind if your hot flashes come with built-in migraines. Table 12.1 lists some common situations that can trigger migraines.

TABLE 12.1: MIGRAINE TRIGGERS

Foods	Body Changes	Environment
Alcohol	Stress	Altitude changes
Some cheeses	Hormonal fluctuations	Weather changes
Chocolate	Physical activity	Time-zone changes
Carob		Air pollution
Caffeine		Bright lights
Citrus		Perfume
Food additives (sodium nitrite, MSG)		

← **Note!**
Three of every four migraine headaches occur in women.

Migraines can be distinguished from other types of headaches by a pulsing, throbbing pain on one side of the head. Sometimes, migraines are accompanied by nausea, pronounced sensitivity to light and sound, and visual disturbances. Always check with your physician if a severe headache involves visual symptoms; those symptoms can indicate an acute problem.

Medicinally induced hot flashes

If you suspect that something else is exacerbating the number of hot flashes you're having, you may be right—and you should definitely discuss it with your doctor. Other medical conditions that can be confused with hot flashes include thyroid disease as well as other rare disorders related to excessive production of endocrine substances. Sometimes certain medications can induce hot flashes.

The FDA has approved several GnRH analogs for treating endometriosis, including leuprolide (Lupron), nafarelin (Synarel), and goserelin (Zoladex). These medicines are structurally similar to the body's own gonadotropin-releasing hormone (GnRH), the hormone that ultimately stimulates estrogen production. Since these drugs are similar to GnRH, they act as decoys, blocking GnRH action which then reduces estrogen levels. Fibroids, which are benign tumors of the uterus, are stimulated by estrogen and often cause excessive bleeding. (More on this topic later in this chapter.) Although these drugs are not specifically approved for use in treating fibroids, such so-called *off-label* use is still considered to be legal and ethical in the medical community. Use of these medicines induces a pseudo or false menopause, which is sometimes helpful to those women experiencing problems from endometriosis or fibroids during their peri-menopausal years.

Other medicines that compete with estrogen also induce hot flashes. Tamoxifen (see Chapter 9), for example, is given to breast cancer patients as well as to women who are at high risk of developing breast cancer. It often induces hot flashes.

Because vasoconstrictors are used to treat hot flashes, it stands to reason that drugs that dilate blood vessels (such as theophylline and nitroglyc-erin) may intensify a hot flash.

Niacin, Vitamin B_3, can also induce hot flashes when taken in large doses. It is often recommended for those at risk of heart disease. A dose of 500 mil-ligrams or more will result in sensations similar to a hot flash.

Vaginal dryness

Vaginal dryness is often one of the first signs of menopause and it is often a very distressing one to many women. The vagina is very sensitive to decreas-ing estrogen levels. As estrogen decreases during late perimenopause, the vagina responds by losing its thickness and elasticity. Lubrication during sex-ual arousal may also decrease. The result is often pain and burning during or after sexual intercourse. Decreased lubrication and elasticity make the vagina more susceptible to trauma during sex. Sometimes a vicious cycle develops in which sex causes irritation, which causes pain, which causes anxiety, which causes inability to lubricate, which causes even more irritation. For many women (and for their partners) this can be a distressing situation. Not only do many women have doubts about their changing libido, but to add insult to injury (and often it may seem as though they *are* injured) a once pleasurable activity is now associated with discomfort.

In addition to physical changes that occur in the vagina, the normal vaginal mixture of bacteria (called the bacterial flora) found prior to menopause undergoes a change. Estrogen normally helps to maintain a mix of different bacteria with a predominance of a type of bacteria called lactobacilli. These healthy lactobacilli help to maintain the proper pH (the balance of acidity) and prevent less healthy bacteria as well as yeast from overgrowing. A very common bacterial infection is called bacterial vaginosis (BV). BV occurs when less favorable bacteria predominate. The end result of vaginal thinning and bacterial flora changes is often a vagina that is more prone to irritation. The resultant condition, called atrophic vaginitis, is characterized by vaginal irritation and watery discharge.

So, what is a sexually active menopausal woman with vaginal irritation to do? If the cause of vaginal discomfort is unknown, a pelvic exam is the first step. Therapy can then be geared to the specific problem. BV is best treated with antibiotics; yeast with antifungal agents. Other potential causes of vaginal discomfort include lacerations or tears due to traumatic intercourse. If atrophic vaginitis is the root of the problem, then a short course of vaginal estrogens can be very beneficial until healing has occurred. Once the vagina is healed and back to baseline then estrogen can be stopped and other measures can be taken to avoid irritation without further hormone use.

The best tactic is to avoid irritation in the first place. When having sexual intercourse, use a lubricant if your own natural lubrication is not sufficient. There are many new products on the market. Liquid lubricants such as AstroGlide and K-Y Liquid (not to be confused with K-Y Jelly) are improvements over older jelly products, since they are more like natural fluids. Other options are vaginal moisturizers. These are nonhormonal products inserted into the vagina several times per week independent of sexual activity. The moisturizers adhere to the vaginal walls and provide more continuous lubrication. Some good products are GyneMoistrin, K-Y Long Lasting, and Replens. All these products are available over the counter without prescription.

Frequent intercourse is also helpful. The phrase "use it or lose it" pertains to vaginal tone and health. Sexual activity increases blood flow to the vagina, and this in turn helps nourish the vagina.

Finally, if you're not in a monogamous relationship, don't hesitate to use condoms. Menopausal women, especially those not using HRT, have thinner vaginal walls that are more susceptible to breaks and tears during intercourse. This of course is a prime way for the AIDS virus to be transmitted. Don't leave yourself open to this infection!

Irregular bleeding and related problems

As hormone levels run askew during peri-menopause and throughout menopause itself, some women's periods seem to take on a life of their own, lasting two or three times as long as usual or occurring as excessively heavy bleeding. Some unfortunate women suffer with periods that are both prolonged and heavy.

Abnormal bleeding can be the result of several factors, and often more than one factor is responsible. Factors responsible for abnormal bleeding include the following:

▪ Hormone changes: During perimenopause, hormone levels become erratic. As explained in Chapter 4, normal ovulatory menstrual cycles are characterized by a predictable rise and fall of estrogen and progesterone. During peri-menopause hormonal imbalances result when ovulation fails to occur on schedule. This often results in abnormal bleeding.

▪ Structural abnormalities: Endometrial polyps are small benign growths arising from the inner lining of the uterus. Fibroids (also called myomas) occur in 30 to 40 percent of women over the age of 30. They grow in the wall of the uterus. Depending on their location in the uterus as well as their size, they can cause problems such as bleeding or discomfort. Fibroids that bulge into the inner cavity of the uterus tend to cause the most significant bleeding problems. Fibroids that are large may cause discomfort due to pressure exerted on the bladder or lower back.

Unofficially... Excessively heavy bleeding that occurs at the expected time of a menstrual period is called menorrhagia. Bleeding that occurs at a time other than the expected menstrual period is called metrorrhagia. Menometrorrhagia is a combination of the two conditions.

- Malignancy: Endometrial cancer (cancer from the inner lining of the uterus), cervical cancer (cancer from the cervix, or mouth of the uterus), and sarcoma (cancer arising from the wall of the uterus) are the types of cancer that can occur in the uterus. They can all cause abnormal bleeding.

- Pregnancy: This is less likely to occur in the late perimenopause, but it is a diagnosis to be considered whenever abnormal bleeding occurs. Although rare, pregnancy is possible up until one year from the time of a last period. Alternatively, a blood test that reveals elevated levels of *both* FSH and LH is a good indication that pregnancy will not occur.

Proper management of abnormal bleeding depends on accurate diagnosis of the cause of bleeding. A menstrual history detailing times of abnormal bleeding as well as any associated events is very helpful. Abnormalities to note and report to your doctor are as follows:

- A change in your regular monthly bleeding pattern
- Bleeding between periods
- Abnormally heavy bleeding with clots
- Frequent bleeding (bleeding that occurs more than every three weeks)
- Bleeding that occurs after intercourse
- Bleeding that occurs after more than one year's absence of a period

Based on this information, tests can be performed to determine the cause of abnormal bleeding. If pregnancy is a possibility, a pregnancy test should be done.

Cancer as a cause of abnormal bleeding

The exclusion of cancer is the next priority. PAP smears of the cervix should be performed on a regular basis to screen for cervical cancer. Endometrial cancer (cancer that occurs in the lining of the uterus) is most often screened with an office procedure called an endometrial biopsy. During this procedure your doctor threads a thin, flexible tubular device through the opening of the cervix into the uterine cavity. Gentle suction is then created, and cells from the endometrial lining are aspirated and sent to the pathology lab where they are evaluated microscopically. The entire procedure takes less than 10 minutes and usually involves mild cramping that resolves quickly. Pre-medication with ibuprofen is helpful. An anesthetic can be injected into the cervix at your doctor's discretion. Endometrial biopsy evaluates abnormal bleeding in much the same way as dilation and curettage (D&C). D&C is indicated if the endometrial biopsy cannot be performed due to technical difficulties or if it is inconclusive. Both tests can determine if there are any cancerous or pre-cancerous cells present. In addition, the pathologist will often make an assessment of the presence or absence of estrogen and progesterone in the endometrial lining. This can be helpful to your physician in evaluating your hormonal status as part of the investigation for abnormal bleeding.

Another helpful tool in evaluating abnormal bleeding is the transvaginal sonogram. (The term "ultrasound" is synonymous with "sonogram.") In this test a thin probe with a sonogram source at the tip is inserted into the vagina. Sound waves are bounced from the probe to your pelvic structures and then back to the probe. An image of your pelvic organs is displayed on a screen, and the endometrial lining can be evaluated for thickness and signs of irregular masses. An endometrial lining thickness of less than 5 millimeters is rarely associated with endometrial cancer or its precursors.

Sarcoma is a rare malignancy arising from the wall of the uterus. Uterine masses that grow at unexpected rates, especially in menopausal women, should be suspected for this cancer. Ovarian cancer does not typically present as abnormal bleeding, and unfortunately this malignancy is much more difficult to detect. Diagnosis of ovarian cancer is made via pelvic exam, sonogram, and ultimately surgical removal of the ovary.

Endometrial cancer (cancer from the lining of the uterus) is by far the most common type of uterine cancer. If anything positive can be said about this malignancy, it is that abnormal bleeding is a symptom that usually leads to early diagnosis. When it is diagnosed in its early stages, this cancer has an excellent prognosis, with over 95 percent survival.

Diagnosis of structural abnormalities

Once malignancy has been ruled out, evaluation for structural abnormalities such as benign polyps and fibroids should be performed. These growths, as mentioned earlier, are extremely common in perimenopausal and menopausal women. Polyps are small (usually less than an inch in size) growths attached to the uterus or cervix by a narrow stalk. They appear in the cervix as well as the endometrial lining. Polyps arising from the cervix are common and almost always benign. They are easily seen on routine pelvic exam and can be easily and painlessly removed in the office. Polyps arising in the endometrial lining can be detected and treated, as we'll discuss below.

Fibroids (myomas) arise from the muscular wall of the uterus. They are round, firm growths that vary in size from small (less than an inch) to large (sometimes 9 or 10 inches or even larger). Often there are more than one fibroid present, so it is not so much the size of each individual fibroid but the sum and total of their mass effect that is responsible for problems. Fibroids may be located within the wall of the uterus (intramural), bulging into the uterine cavity (submucous), protruding from the outside of the uterus (subserosal), or attached on a thin base (pedunculated). The location and size of the fibroid often determines the type and severity of symptoms. Bleeding problems are most prevalent with submucous fibroids and with large intramural fibroids. These types increase the total surface area of the uterine cavity, presenting the endometrial lining with a larger volume of material to be shed. In addition, the lining becomes stretched and attenuated over these bulging masses, which prevents the body's normal mechanisms that stop bleeding from kicking in. These fibroids typically produce the annoying symptoms of menometrorrhagia—that is, heavy periods as well as bleeding in between periods. Often it is not until perimenopause, when hormonal fluctuations start, that fibroids present with bleeding problems.

Although fibroids can usually be detected during a routine pelvic exam, a sonogram may be needed to determine whether they are distorting the uterine cavity. Pelvic sonograms can be performed in one of several ways. Originally sonograms were performed with the transducer (the instrument that sends out the ultrasound waves) applied to the skin of the lower abdomen. This technique gives an excellent overview of the pelvic organs but does not allow as much detail of the uterus and ovaries as does the transvaginal approach described earlier. Transvaginal sonograms give us more information about the thickness of the endometrial lining as well as the presence of possible fibroids, polyps, or masses. A new technique to further evaluate the uterine cavity is called a sonohysterogram. Sterile water is introduced through a small tube placed in the cervix. While the water fills the cavity of the uterus, a transvaginal sonogram is performed. This allows excellent visualization of structures and masses protruding into the cavity and can determine whether or not structural defects are a potential source of bleeding. It can also delineate whether or not an abnormality seen on a transvaginal sonogram is due to a polyp or a thickened lining.

Other techniques are at your gynecologist's disposal to evaluate structural problems. An X-ray test called a hysterosalpingogram (HSG) follows the same principle as the sonohystergram. In a similar fashion, X-ray dye is injected into the uterus while X-ray pictures are taken. Some doctors prefer this test to the sonogram version. Another way to evaluate the endometrial cavity is to take a direct look. This can be accomplished with hysteroscopy. In this procedure a diagnostic scope is inserted through the cervix and into the cavity. Visualization of the cavity then becomes possible. This procedure can be performed in the office or in the operating room, with the decision based on the extent of the procedure to be performed, your medical condition, and your physician's capabilities.

Treatment of abnormal bleeding with medications

Today there are many options available to the peri-menopausal woman with abnormal bleeding. Hysterectomy is no longer the knee-jerk response that it once was to this problem, although sometimes it still is the best answer. The key is to determine what is causing the abnormal bleeding and then to follow a treatment plan that best suits the individual woman's needs.

Once malignancy is ruled out of the picture, some women opt to do nothing at all. This is appropriate as long as the bleeding is mild and there are other reasonable explanations for the abnormal bleeding (such as perimenopausal hormone fluctuations or fibroid tumors). In those cases, an iron supplement should be taken and periodic blood counts should be performed to check for anemia. The situation can always be reevaluated if it worsens.

Other perimenopausal women may find abnormal bleeding unacceptable. They may not be symptomatic enough for surgical intervention or may only be bothered by bleeding irregularities due to hormonal fluctuations. Low dose oral contraceptive (OC) pills may be a good option for these women. These pills have the lowest dose of estrogen available, 20 micrograms of ethinyl estradiol, compared to the 30 to 35 microgram doses of other OCs. Some pills in this category (at the time of this writing) are Mircette, LoEstrin 1/20, and Alesse. Women who smoke, have breast cancer, unexplained vaginal bleeding, history of blood clots, as well as other medical conditions that may have prevented them from taking OCs in the past are not candidates for these pills. Benefits of low dose OCs include the following:

Watch Out!
Another cause of heavy vaginal bleeding is a condition called adenomyosis, in which the endometrial lining grows *into* the muscular wall of the uterus. Periods typically are heavy and very painful. Endometrial biopsy and sono-grams are unreliable diagnostic tools—the only true way to diagnose it is when a hysterectomy is performed and the uterus is examined by the pathologist.

- Excellent contraception during a phase when unintended pregnancy can occur
- Elimination of bleeding between periods
- Decrease in the amount of monthly bleeding
- Elimination of dysmenorrhea (painful periods)
- Periods that are predictable
- Elimination of hot flashes, insomnia, vaginal dryness, and mood fluctuations

Many times, use of low dose OCs is all that's needed to help a woman through her perimenopausal transition. If this route is taken, the pill should be periodically discontinued in order to re-evaluate for the presence of menopause (by testing for FSH and LH), and thus the indication that OCs should be permanently discontinued. If both FSH and LH are elevated, then the likelihood of pregnancy is low, as is occasional ovulation, and OCs should be stopped.

There are other medications that can be used to treat abnormal bleeding, although only for limited intervals of time. As mentioned earlier in this chapter the group of GnRH analogs (Lupron, Synarel, and Zoladex) can be used to decrease estrogen levels as a means of stopping uterine bleeding. This is usually used as a way to stop excessively heavy bleeding prior to performing a surgical treatment. These medications are indicated only for short-term use (up to six months) and are costly. The advantage is that they may allow a woman to reverse anemia, thus avoiding a blood transfusion prior to surgery. In selected cases they can stop bleeding so that uterine conserving surgery (see below) may be more easily performed.

Treatment of abnormal bleeding with surgery

Over the last two decades there has been an explosion of surgical options available to the gynecologist. Twenty years ago most women over the age of 40 with excessive bleeding would almost certainly undergo a hysterectomy. Today that trend has reversed due to pressure from public interest groups as well as the availability of new treatment modalities. The decision to undergo surgery (except in cases of malignancy when surgery is usually the preferred treatment) is often a choice made by a woman when her symptoms become too annoying to tolerate. The type of procedure performed depends on the origin of the problem, the surgeon's skill, and the individual's desires once the risks and benefits of these procedures are explored. While there is a growing trend towards avoiding hysterectomy, there is no doubt that in certain cases it is still the best procedure. However, as is the case with any surgical procedure, don't go into it lightly, and make sure you thoroughly understand all potential risks and benefits. Before undergoing any procedure you should feel satisfied that all your questions have been addressed. If not, don't hesitate to seek out another opinion.

Advances in hysteroscopy have allowed a whole new approach to treating structural problems affecting the uterine cavity. As mentioned above, hysteroscopy involves inserting an instrument into the uterine cavity, which then allows the gynecologist to visualize the inner surface of the uterus. New scopes also allow introduction of instruments that can excise, grasp, burn, and remove structures. Office hysteroscopy can be performed with minimal use of pain medicines. It is most useful in removing small polyps. More extensive procedures should be done in the operating room. The following procedures can be performed with the hysteroscope in the operating room:

- *Polypectomy:* Relatively larger polyps should be removed in the operating room due to the risk of heavy bleeding and the need for anesthesia.

- *Myomectomy:* This procedure involves the removal of only the fibroid, without removing the uterus. This approach is particularly useful when there is a solitary submucous fibroid bulging into the uterine cavity. Many times it is necessary to pre-treat with a GnRH analogue in order to decrease bleeding as well as the size of the fibroid. The fibroid is removed as close to its base as possible using an attachment called a resectascope, which uses an electric current to help with the excision. Potential complications include excessive bleeding, damage to internal organs, and—rarely—fluid overload that can result in fatal congestive heart failure. There is also the possibility that the fibroid can grow back over time. When this technique is used in the properly selected patient, the results are very satisfying. It can resolve an annoying problem with a minimally invasive procedure.

- *Endometrial Ablation:* This technique uses either the resectascope mentioned above or an attachment called a rollerball. Both techniques involve destruction of the endometrial lining via an electric current that is applied over the surface of the uterine cavity. By destroying the endometrial lining, the portion of the uterus that actually bleeds becomes nonfunctional. The challenge is to destroy enough of the lining so that a decrease in bleeding actually occurs.

Because it is difficult, if not impossible, to destroy the entire lining with this technique, results are variable. One third of women experience no change in bleeding, one third have improvement, and one third have complete cessation of bleeding. Risks are similar to those of hysteroscopic myomectomy.

ThermaChoice Uterine Balloon Therapy is a similar technique that actually doesn't require a hysteroscope, but instead uses a patented instrument made by Ethicon. In this procedure the instrument is inserted into the uterus, a balloonlike apparatus is inflated inside the cavity, and heat is delivered to the uterine lining in sufficient amounts to destroy it. Since the technique is not suitable for use in a fibroid uterus, it has limited application at this time, although it appears to have great potential.

Short of doing a hysterectomy (discussed below), another surgical treatment is myomectomy performed from the abdominal route, that is, via an incision into the abdominal wall. In this operation fibroids (also called myomas) are removed, and the uterus is reconstructed and left in place. The advantage is that the uterus can be preserved while the problem parts are removed. (Some people would argue that this is in fact a *disadvantage* since the woman is now left with a nonfunctioning organ that can only potentially cause bleeding or develop cancer.) When considering a myomectomy the potential risks should be considered:

■ There is generally a greater potential for excessive blood loss during this operation. Look into banking your own blood prior to undergoing this procedure to decrease the risk of receiving a blood transfusion from a donor.

- There is always the chance that fibroids can grow back. Whatever process caused you to develop fibroids in the first place may allow you to develop new ones in the future.

- If you decide to go on HRT after your surgery, you may experience annoying bleeding. You will also have to take a progestin along with estrogen.

All in all, this is a procedure that usually has excellent results, especially when done in the peri-menopausal phase when regrowth of myomas is less likely to occur than during the reproductive phase of life. (Successful outcomes are also more likely when the uterus is on the smaller side, with large fibroids making it a trickier procedure to perform.) Many women fear their sexual response or bladder function may change when a hysterectomy is performed and opt for this organ preserving operation instead.

Hysterectomy is the surgical removal of the uterus. There are many different types of hysterectomy:

- Total abdominal hysterectomy is the removal of the uterus and cervix through an abdominal incision. (Note that this does not include removal of the ovaries, which we'll discuss later.) This is the operation of choice for those women with large fibroids, who have had a previous myomectomy, who don't want to have future bleeding, or who don't want to take a progestin during HRT. If the uterus is large (roughly the size of a 4 to 5 month pregnant uterus), it may be less traumatic to undergo hysterectomy than myomectomy, which requires healing of the retained uterus.

- Supracervical hysterectomy is the removal of the uterus, leaving the cervix behind. This procedure is done in difficult surgical cases in which removal of the cervix may lead to trauma of the bladder or in those surgeries in which the patient is too unstable to allow time for removal of the cervix. There is a growing trend amongst women to request this procedure in the hope of having less distortion to the vagina and bladder, changes that *may* affect sexuality and bladder control. If this procedure is performed and if HRT is used, it is important to add a progestin to the regimen since the remaining cervix has the capacity to respond in the same manner as endometrial tissue.

- Vaginal hysterectomy is the surgical removal of the uterus and cervix through the vagina, thus avoiding an abdominal scar. These procedures are most commonly performed for a prolapsed uterus, a situation in which the uterus protrudes through the vagina due to weakened support. It is best performed on a small uterus, although certain gynecologists have skill in removing even a very large fibroid uterus via this approach. The advantage is a shorter and easier recovery.

- Laparoscopic assisted vaginal hysterectomy (LAVH) is surgical removal of the uterus and cervix using a new technique that combines laparoscopic surgery (surgery performed with operating scopes placed into the abdomen through tiny incisions) with vaginal removal of the uterus. In this operation laparoscopic surgery is used to free the upper portion of the uterus via laparoscopic instruments inserted through several small incisions in the abdominal wall. Once this is accomplished the remainder of the hysterectomy is performed in a similar fashion to vaginal hysterectomy. This procedure allows vaginal removal of a uterus that would have previously been possible only via the abdominal route. The benefit is faster recovery since the abdominal scars are very small.

When it comes to hysterectomy in a perimenopausal or menopausal woman, the issue of whether or not to remove the ovaries must be discussed. In the past, it was very clear-cut: Those women 45 years or older were advised to have bilateral salpingo-oophorectomy (BSO), or removal of both ovaries. Women between the ages of 40 and 45 were counseled, but ultimately were given the choice of whether or not to do a BSO. The reasoning was that menopause was imminent, and with it the ovaries became useless organs that were only at risk of developing cancer. While ovarian cancer is still the most deadly gynecologic malignancy, there is also the realization that perimenopausal and early menopausal ovaries still produce androgens. Any woman undergoing hysterectomy should weigh the pros and cons of BSO and relate them to her own particular situation.

A new, cutting-edge procedure to treat fibroids is called selective embolization. It works on the following principle: If the blood supply to a fibroid can be compromised, that fibroid will shrink. The procedure is performed by a radiologist who starts by doing an angiogram of the pelvic arteries. In this procedure thin catheters are guided (via X-ray technology) into the blood vessels that nourish the most troublesome fibroids. Medication that forms a clot is then injected directly into the blood vessels in question. (The process of sending off a clot is called embolization.) The procedure is very new and not in wide use. It requires a high degree of skill and is costly. The process can be painful as well, since the fibroid in question must die off from lack of blood flow, not dissimilar to the situation that occurs in a heart attack. On the other hand, it has the benefit of removing fibroid tumors without any surgical scars. It is a technique to watch.

Surgical interventions for hormone problems

Although a complete hysterectomy can certainly resolve severe problems in a perimenopausal woman, it also induces menopause and therefore is known as *surgical menopause*. When the ovaries are removed, the body's main source of estrogen production is no longer available, and hormone-replacement therapy is usually recommended.

Even after hysterectomy alone (without removal of the ovaries), women tend to enter menopause as much as four years earlier than they might have if surgery had not been done, according to one study.

More than half a million hysterectomies are performed every year in the United States. Due to criticism from patient advocacy groups over the last decade, there has been a growing trend to treat the problems that once resulted in hysterectomy and ovary removal with less invasive treatments. Although some women sail through hysterectomy and ovary removal with ideal results, others experience continuing hormonal problems or never feel quite like themselves.

A third of all hysterectomies are performed for conditions that involve uterine fibroids, which can

Watch Out!
The suggestion that you no longer need your ovaries or your uterus should bring a response of healthy skepticism and a determination to get a second (and, preferably, third) opinion. If your medical situation is serious enough to warrant hysterectomy, so be it; but do not go into this or *any* surgery without a thorough discussion with your doctors about risks, benefits, and alternative treatments.

Bright Idea
The HERS
(Hysterectomy
Educational
Resource and
Services)
Foundation is a
not-for-profit
entity that can
assist you in
obtaining more
information on
this operation.
Contact HERS at
422 Bryn Mawr
Avenue, Bala
Cynwyd, PA
19004, (610)
667-7757. The
fax number is
(610) 667-8096,
and the e-mail
address is
hersFDN@
aol.com.

cause heavy bleeding and pain. Some surgical alternatives to hysterectomy are available in many situations, however.

Some life-threatening conditions can warrant hysterectomy, but the operation is often performed for reasons that are *not* life-threatening. People who are critical of the practice make the following points:

- Women may experience a loss of sexual sensation as a result of hysterectomy.

- There may be displacement of the bladder or intestines, which in turn can lead to incontinence or digestive disorders.

- Hormonal production is thwarted when reproductive organs are removed, increasing reliance on outside sources of hormones (HRT).

Decisions, decisions: handling menopause your way

No matter what your age or current experience with menopause or perimenopause, you can benefit by taking care of yourself: getting good nutrition, getting adequate exercise, and keeping stress at bay. The earlier you begin a health regimen, the better off you'll be later, when you may really need the help.

We hope that this chapter is the beginning of your exploration of ways to better your health and prevent illness. Whether you decide to take a conventional route with regard to replacement therapy or seek to stabilize your hormones by using herbs and other alternative methods, please remember that your health and happiness are your responsibility, which is a serious one.

Seek the advice of a good physician (make sure that you have a good physician), and don't ever be afraid to solicit a second opinion. Take part in your own medical care by keeping yourself informed. Learn how to do a little research on your own, and find a community of other women who have some of the same concerns so that you can compare notes—online, via a mailing list or newsgroup; in a support group that meets once a month; or informally, among your network of friends. Menopause is a step in maturity. You can rise to the occasion and handle it beautifully by actively seeking out the best advice *and* thinking for yourself.

Just the facts

- Antihypertensive medications such as Clonidine can be helpful in relieving hot flashes.

- Some prescription medicines can intensify hot flashes.

- Vaginal dryness can be managed with a variety of nonhormonal lubricant products.

- There are many new options, both medical and surgical, available to women with abnormal perimenopausal bleeding.

Alternatives and Environmental Issues

PART V

GET THE SCOOP ON...
Western, Chinese, and Indian herbs that may
aid your hormones ▪ Acupuncture, shiatsu, and
other hands-on treatments ▪
Whether herbs are really safe to use ▪ How
homeopathy is used for menopause

Herbs and Alternative Treatments

Chapter 13

For centuries, humans have relied on herbs for medicinal needs, and most of the world's population still relies on herbs in health care. The development of specific drugs for treating illness is a fairly recent occurrence. Should the advent of pharmaceuticals outmode herbal remedies? Are modern medicines better?

Sales of herbal medicine in the United States top $1.5 billion annually and are on the rise. Clearly, plenty of people are willing to give herbs a go. Traditional Asian medicine—with its patent herbal medicines, acupuncture, shiatsu massage, and Ayurvedic Indian regimens (which concentrate on herbs and foods)—are undergoing a resurgence in popularity. Homeopathy is also among the alternative approaches that work for many women. Each form of therapy has its critics, but so does pharmaceutical-based Western medicine.

This chapter introduces some of the most popular herbs and formulas used for menopause. The chapter also provides a short course on the philosophies behind various alternative menopause therapies.

Effective herbalism?

What do you know about herbs? Aside from flavoring food, do they do any good for illnesses? Now may be a good time to examine your biases (if you have any) about herbal therapies; you could be in for a surprise. Quiz 13.1 is a quick way to check what you know—and what you don't.

QUIZ 13.1: HOW'S YOUR HERB KNOWLEDGE?

True	False	
☐	☐	1. When you use herbs, you're relying on folklore and word of mouth, rather than on hard evidence about their effects.
☐	☐	2. Herbs can be a better approach to menopause because they're natural and, therefore, safe, whereas the drugs or hormones that your doctor prescribes may not be.
☐	☐	3. Most of the world relies on pharmaceuticals instead of herbs for medicine because pharmaceuticals simply work better.
☐	☐	4. As long as you take a decent vitamin supplement, you don't need herbs to help with difficult menopausal or perimenopausal symptoms.
☐	☐	5. Herbs may help flavor my food, but they're not going to do anything for my hormones (although maybe St. John's wort will help my mood).

Answers: An astute herbalist knows that the answer to all these questions is False.

Yes, herbs can work. But they're not always safe just because they're natural. Plenty of plants out there in the wild would have no problem killing you, or at least making you ill, if you ate them. Remember your last brush with poison ivy? Enough said.

One of the comforts of using pharmaceuticals is that they seem to be known commodities, with tested effects, so you *are* relying on evidence rather than folklore. But do we have a fighting chance of ever knowing the mechanism of the action of a specific herb—or whether it has any action at all? Absolutely.

Although herbs have not necessarily gone through years of animal and human testing before hitting the market place, traditional double-blind clinical tests and lab studies are often performed on popular herbs, and some have a good deal of research backing them up.

There is medical evidence to support the estrogenic activity of herbs as well as their potential anti-cancer effects. The estrogen effects of herbs are not as potent, for the most part, as traditional HRT.

There is, however, medical information to support claims that herbal estrogen decreases hot flashes and ameliorates mood swings. Some studies show herbal estrogen benefits bone strength and cardiovascular status while it concurrently does not appear to increase breast or endometrial cancer risk. The extent of these actions has yet to be fully explored, and more studies are in the works. Sometimes, however, a little information can be misrepresented. Claims of herbal benefits have been made without full scientific study to back them up. While many women using herbs find relief from hot flashes and mood changes associated with menopause, there is no evidence at this time to support that herbs will benefit bone strength, cardiovascular status, or brain function to the extent that HRT does. As with any medical information, take your herbs with a grain of salt.

Scientific studies show that plant estrogens, called phytoestrogens, are capable of binding to estrogen receptors. It is this activity that gives phytoestrogens their estrogenlike activity as well as their anti-estrogen activity. Black cohosh, for example, has been studied and was found to suppress luteinizing hormone (LH) and to bind to estrogen receptors. (It is marketed under the name Remifemin.) By binding to estrogen receptors, herbal estrogens exert a similar but lesser response than estradiol.

There is growing evidence that some herbs may be potent anticancer agents. Since phytoestrogens are capable of binding to estrogen receptors and act as weak estrogens, they may be able to block the effects of stronger estrogens such as estradiol, which may be associated with stimulating breast and endometrial tumor growth. In this way, weak herbal estrogens may have some estrogen effects (agonist activity) while at the same time blocking estrogen (antagonist activity). More scientific study is in progress to explore this exciting prospect.

How herbs help menopause

What about herbs for menopause? Many popular varieties are available at health food stores and drug stores these days, and prepackaged menopause teas and herbal combination formulas abound.

There is medical evidence to support the estrogenic activity of some herbs as well as their potential anti-cancer effects. The estrogen effects of herbs (as they're traditionally used) can be powerful but are not typically *as* potent as traditional HRT. There is medical information to support claims that herbs containing estrogens decrease hot flashes and ameliorate mood swings. Some studies show they benefit bone strength and cardiovascular status while they concurrently do not *appear* to increase breast or endometrial cancer risk. The extent of these actions has yet to be fully explored, and more studies are in the works.

Claims of herbal benefits have often been made without full scientific study to back them up. And while any lack of studies does not mean that the herbs don't work, bear in mind that you may be relying on anecdotal evidence and hearsay in some cases—there's less data, and sometimes no *strict* data, to rely on.

While many women using herbs find relief from hot flashes and mood changes associated with menopause, it hasn't been established whether herbs will benefit bone strength, cardiovascular status, or brain function *to the extent* that HRT does, or not. As with any medical information, take your herbs with a grain of salt.

Scientific studies show that many plant estrogens, called phytoestrogens, are capable of binding to human estrogen receptors. It is this activity that gives phytoestrogens their estrogenic activity as well as their anti-estrogen activity. When a weak plant estrogen binds to a human estrogen receptor, it can take up that space where otherwise a more powerful human estrogen might bind, thus in the body seeming to *reduce* estrogenicity by providing the less potent form.

Black cohosh, for example, has been studied and was found to suppress luteinizing hormone (LH) and to bind to estrogen receptors. (It is marketed under the name Remifemin.) There are a variety of plant estrogens weaker in activity than human estradiol, though some plants contain hormones identical in structure to human estrogens, *including* estradiol.

There is growing evidence that some herbs may be potent anti-cancer agents. It is because phytoestrogens are capable of binding to estrogen receptors and act as weak estrogens that they may be helpful against cancer through their ability to block the effects of stronger estrogens such as estradiol which may be associated with stimulating breast and endometrial tumor growth. More scientific study is in progress to explore this exciting prospect.

Expect to hear more about the medicinal aspects of herbs from a scientific perspective. It's now possible to fingerprint the chemicals that herbs contain, and as you might imagine, the quantity of constituents can vary, depending on the region where a plant is grown and other conditions. As the active ingredients in herbs are increasingly identified, drug companies' interest in those active ingredients can be expected to increase as well.

A short history of herbs

In the United States, the thought of going to the doctor is associated with the idea of getting a drug prescription. In other countries, the situation is different. Most of the world's population has to rely on herbs for many medical needs. Poverty and unavailability, as well as tradition, keep the use of pharmaceuticals limited.

Bright Idea
Medline allows you to search thousands of medical-journal abstracts on herbs and traditional Chinese medicine, as well as typical Western drugs and conditions. Use your favorite search engine to find a Medline gateway, or try the one at www. healthworld.com.

China, which has a rich medical history spanning thousands of years, is slow to embrace Western medicine, though it is increasingly being adapted for use *alongside* traditional Chinese medicine (TCM), which relies on acupuncture, herbs, and similar therapies. Conversely, in the United States, TCM is gaining popularity.

In tradition-rich Europe, reliance on herbal approaches and homeopathy is greater than in the United States.

But the United States has also made some important contributions to herbs and herbalism. A popular type of mild ginseng that is used worldwide—even in China, the land of ginseng—is American ginseng, which grows wild in Kentucky, Vermont, the Blue Ridge Mountains, and the Catskills.

Hormonal effects from herbs

If you've read about *phytohormones*, (and see Chapter 14 for more details) you know that plants can have hormonal effects in the human body. Soy, for example, has powerful phytoestrogens. Many herbs that have a reputation in folklore and country medicine for helping women's problems are now being analyzed for their chemical components. We know much more about these herbs and their effects today, but people have relied on basic herbal wisdom for ages. Certain herbs were used because of anecdotal proof that they had the desired effects.

Analysis of various botanicals reveals that some have pronounced estrogenic qualities, and different parts of the plant can have different levels of capability. For example, the soybean seed is more potently estrogenic than its leaf. And plants may contain a number of different active chemicals.

Unofficially...
Some countries (Denmark, Germany, and Sweden, to name three) already have restrictive laws about herbal supplements, and those laws could get stricter as new herb guidelines are developed by the World Health Organization and the United Nations. There is discussion of tightening standards in the United States as well.

Some well-known botanicals with particularly high counts of estrogenic agents include:

- Licorice root

- Soybean seed

- Fenugreek seed

- Red clover

- Rhubarb

- Carrot

- Black cumin seed

- Evening primrose seed

- Sage leaf

The estrogenic potency of plants was first discovered in the 1940's when Australian sheep farmers found that ewes that grazed in certain clover pastures became infertile. Further scientific investigation of the clover revealed a high level of phytoestrogens. When the ewes were fed this clover, estrogenic effects were demonstrated in the uterus, and there was a decline in luteinizing hormone (LH) that prevented ovulation.

While some plants are high in the concentration of one estrogenic component, others have a variety. Licorice, for example, is commonly used in both TCM and Western herbalism. That herb contains the following estrogenic chemicals:

- Anethole

- Beta-sitosterol

- Estriol (a human estrogen)

- Genistein

- Glycyrrhizin

- Stigmasterol

Watch Out!
For all its benefits, licorice has been known to promote water retention in a significant number of users. Whenever you're taking herbs, monitor them for unwanted effects, and adjust your herbal plan accordingly.

Being whole foods, herbs often contain opposing substances, and proponents of herb use maintain that such balance helps mediate appropriate actions in the human body—which over history has developed and adapted in response to substances in its natural environment. Licorice, to stick with the preceding example, contains antiestrogens such as the following:

- Apigenin
- Beta-sitosterol (which is also estrogenic)
- Ferulic acid
- Formononetin
- Glycyrrhetic acid
- Glycyrrhizin
- Quercetin

Licorice also contains compounds that promote testosterone. This particular herb has many opposing actions and is traditionally used in Chinese medicine to moderate the effects of other herbs—as a balancing tonic, so to speak.

In traditional Chinese medicine, these chemical components were unknown when the standard combinations of herbs that became patent medicines were developed. The Chinese treated a given condition with a blend of herbs, adding a little of this and a little of that or perhaps subtracting a certain component, until they arrived at a blend that had the desired actions on most patients. For patients who weren't quite the norm, TCM practitioners had the option of continuing to add to or subtract from a formula to moderate its effects appropriately.

Traditional Chinese medicine (TCM) and menopause

In traditional Chinese medicine, everything is considered to be *yin* and *yang* to varying degrees. Herbs, treatments, the foods we eat, and the activities or attitudes we espouse all affect the balance of yin and yang in our bodies. Disharmony of yin and yang leads to illness.

Women are considered somewhat more yin in nature, men more yang. Menopause is known as a state of declining yin. Just some of the many qualities of yin and yang are shown in Table 13.1.

TABLE 13.1: YIN & YANG CHARACTERISTICS

Yin	Yang
inner	outer
female	male
cold	hot
negative	positive
still	active
chronic	acute
wet	dry
conserving	outgoing
creation	heaven
blood	energy (Qi)
night	day

When classic problems of menopause occur, they're thought of as consituting the menopausal syndrome Jue Jing Qian Hou Zhu Zhang. Hot flashes, irritability, and some other familiar complaints are very yang in nature. The Chinese say that they happen because the kidney yin has declined to the point that it can no longer adequately control or balance the raging yang.

66
Chinese medicine refers to things—the kidney, the spleen, the heart, the liver— not so much out of an interest in the object or organ itself, but as a group of functions and associations to do with the organ systems and their energy. So when we talk about them, it's very much different than only focusing on the organs."
—Steve Given LAC, Dean of Clinical Education, Yo San University (Santa Monica, CA)
99

In traditional Chinese medicine, the arrival of menopause can be called Jing Duan (menses stopping) or Jue Jing (ending menses), or the cessation of the moon flow (which is described as Tian Gui, "heavenly water" or "heavenly cycle"). The blood for menstruation is thought to be created out of *Jing* (essential energy) from the kidney and the spleen-stomach.

When kidney Jing, affected by declining Yin, can no longer support the monthly loss of menstrual blood (itself a Yin substance), the flow is shut off so that the vital Jing is conserved. This is menopause. For some women this conservation works well, but others develop a chronic deficiency of Jing and blood (not the same as a blood deficiency in Western terms). Chinese herbs are used to restore the deficient Jing and blood.

The Chinese recognized early on just how much a woman's monthly cycle affects her well-being, and in their medical parlance it is said that men are ruled by *Qi* (a type of energy—of course *Yang*) but women are ruled by *blood* (which is *Yin*). With this philosophy, medical practitioners address treatment with an eye toward enriching and balancing the blood—many conditions affecting women are thought of as problems of *depletion*. Care is taken to build, not overstimulate with energetic (Yang) herbs.

Traditional Chinese medicine has been in existence for thousands of years, so it brings a rich history of herbal use to the table. There are volumes of specifics on the nuances of endocrinology and gynecology among the 30,000 medicinal texts comprising its scope. Following are some of the benefits of using TCM therapies during menopause:

- TCM treatment addresses what is believed to be the root cause of health problems, rather than seeking to just help outward symptoms.

- TCM emphasizes making slight adjustments as needed (ideal for complex hormone issues involving feedback systems and balance).

- TCM is an established form of treatment, with much data and anecdotal evidence to back it up.

- Herbs used in TCM may have desirable actions that Western pharmaceuticals do not.

Many of the herbs used in TCM are of a *tonic* or *adaptogenic* nature, which means that they are reputed to enhance balance and to help the body adjust to changes and deal with problems. TCM can also be affordable. In addition, the formulas and herbs used are widely available.

TCM herbal gynecology

Watch Out!
Although you can get herbs and TCM formulas without a physician's prescription, diagnosis and treatment can be complex. To get started on the right track, consult an acupuncturist or a holistic physician who is trained in Chinese medicine.

Three classes of herbs are used in TCM: superior, general, and inferior. The most popular vitalizing herbs belong to the *superior* class of tonic herbs. These herbs are thought to enhance longevity, energy, and the body's ability to handle stress and regulate itself. The second of three classes of herbs is the *general* class of balancing herbs, which are part tonics and part remedies. The goal of these herbs is to normalize body function. Many treatments for menopause-related symptoms fall into the first two classes of herbs.

The third class of herbs—the *inferior* class—consists of herbal remedies, which are geared toward fixing acute problems and are usually used for a short period. The herbs in this class provide counter-attacks for serious illnesses that cannot be remedied by the balancing and tonifying actions of the other two classes of herbs, and their prescribing is best left only to doctors of TCM.

Following are some of the herbs that are frequently recommended for complaints of a female nature:

> **Peony** (called tree peony, paeonia suffruticosa, or Mu Dan Pi). For menstrual disorders, the bark is combined with bupleurum and Dang Quai, and for period cramping it is combined with cinnamon and walnut. It is used to help with typical menopausal complaints such as hot flashes.

> **Bupleurum** (called bupleurum chinense, Chai Hu, or thorowax). Bupleurum is a balancing herb for the female hormones. It is often used to address hot flashes and other menopausal complaints.

> **Dong Quai** (called Tang Kuei, Dang Gui, angelica sinensis, and Chinese angelica). Perhaps the most popular tonic for female reproductive function, Dong Quai can be estrogenic.

> **Cornelian Asiatic cherry** (called Shan Zhu Yu or cornus officinalis). This herb is used to treat abnormally heavy menstruation.

> **Chinese foxglove** (also called Shu Di Huang or rehmania glutinosa). The root of this plant is used to warm the blood. When dried (and typically fried in rice wine), the root is used for menstrual disorders, to combat weakness and restore blood.

> **Dodder seeds** (also called Tu Si Zi and cuscuta chinensis). This herb is used to treat the

Timesaver
Where can you find TCM formulas and herbs? Some herbs, such as Dong Quai, have gone mainstream and may be available at your corner drugstore. A health-food store is an option for harder-to-find herbs, and the definitive source for herb information is your local acupuncturist.

condition known as yang deficiency of the kidney. It is also used to prevent miscarriages and regulate the menstrual cycle.

Following are some patent medicines (premixed formulas) that are used for menopause problems:

To Jing Wan (Regulate the Menses pill). This compound frees stagnant blood, stimulates circulation, and relieves pain. Women who suffer clots, cramping, and irregular periods may benefit from it.

Yun Nan Bai Yao (Yunnan Paiyao). This patent formula is often used to treat traumatic injuries. It stops bleeding, disperses stagnant blood, has a toning effect, and reduces pain. Women use it for excessive menstrual bleeding and cramps.

Yun Nan Te Chan Tian Qi Pian. This formula is often used after the birth of a child to prevent blood stagnation, and it may be best used by women with a tendency toward coldness (literally low body temperature or cold extremities and slow, lethargic movement. The formula has a reputation for warming and activating the circulation, as well as for dispersing clots, halting bleeding, relieving pain, and reducing swelling. It is also used to treat hot flashes and other frequent menopausal difficulties.

Wu Ji Bai Feng Wan (Black Chicken, White Phoenix pill). This formula is a blood tonic and energy-regulation compound that is said to warm the uterus, nourish the yin, and resolve stagnant energy in the liver and blood. Consequently, the formula is used for what in Chinese medicine are known as *cold* or *deficiency* conditions: amenorrhea, dysmenorrhea, and infertility. It is also helpful for fatigue and premenstrual syndrome (PMS).

Pai Feng herbal drops (White Phoenix pill). Pai Feng is a blood- and energy-nourishing formula that is used for conditions similar to those for which Wu Ji Bai Feng Wan is used.

Bu Xue Tiao Jing Pian. This formula is also used for deficiency conditions that involve fatigue, excessive bleeding, cramps, or irregular periods.

Avoiding unwanted effects

As mentioned earlier, traditional Chinese medicine holds that men are ruled by *Qi* and that women are ruled by blood. What does this distinction mean to you? Herbs that are very yang (loosely translated, warming) can be inappropriate for the balance of a woman's system. In TCM, a strongly warming ginseng may be used in an herbal formula for men, but Dong Quai may be used for women instead. (Dong Quai is often referred to as *women's ginseng*, in fact.) You may want to experiment with herbs such as Dong Quai or, if using ginsengs, the cooler varieties (such as American ginseng) to get the effect that you want.

One reason to be careful with ginseng is fluid balance. If you have a tendency to retain water, yang tonics may be the wrong prescription. Ginseng's classical uses include restoring vital energy (*Qi*) and generating fluids, and fluid generation may not be what you're looking for. Similar problems can occur with certain other herbs for some women.

According to Western medicine, the problem with licorice and water retention involves salt. Some

Unofficially...
Some herbs in TCM are used to moderate or counter the actions of other herbs. The presence of licorice in a formula, for example, doesn't necessarily mean that you'll gain water weight. Some of the most popular weight-and-water-loss teas include licorice, but combine it alongside herbal diuretics that might be too strong on their own. The idea is balance.

licorice contains glycyrrhetic acid, which can lead to problems in transforming cortisol to cortisone. That situation prompts the body to increase serum sodium while decreasing serum potassium. The results are water retention and weight increase (and sometimes hypertension) in some women.

A 1996 report in a Dutch medical journal reports the story of a 38-year-old woman who was hospitalized for hypertension and hypokalaemic alkalosis. Her ingestion of 200 grams of licorice daily was found to be the cause. [Seelen MA; de Meijer PH; Braun J; Swinkels LM; Waanders H; Meinders AE; Meijer PH [corrected to de Meijer PH]; Academisch Ziekenhuis, afd. Interne Geneeskunde, Leiden; [Hypertension caused by licorice consumption (published erratum appears in Ned Tijdschr Geneeskd 1997 Jan 18;141(3):176)]; Ned Tijdschr Geneeskd, 140(52):2632-5 1996 Dec 28.]

Some licorice supplements have glycyrrhetic acid removed, however; and herbal proponents suggest that preparations made from whole licorice are less likely to offend than are strong extracts containing the acid.

Ginsengs

There are several varieties of what we call *ginseng*, which is called *ren shen* (man root) in Chinese. Some ginsengs are actually different plants, grouped under the heading ginseng because they have somewhat similar effects. True ginsengs contain compounds called *ginsenosides*, which is where much of their potency lies.

Ginsenosides are similar in structure to the human body's own steroid hormones, but studies suggest that rather than having direct hormonal action, they affect the production of our own hormones. Different ginsengs have different ginsenosides, many of which have been identified. *Panax* ginseng and *tien-chi* ginseng have at least 10 ginsenosides, and *eleuthero* ginseng has at least 7.

More than 20 years ago, research showed that ginseng can relieve stress on the adrenal glands. In recent studies at Jianxi Medical College (in Nanchang, in China's Jianxi province), it was found to affect luteinizing hormone (LH). A similar result has been reported for deer antler, which is often used in combination with ginseng in Chinese formulas. When ginsenosides or active portions of deer antler were administered to lab animals, LH secretion from the pituitary rose about tenfold (as you may recall from Chapter 4, LH has a potent effect on the menstrual cycle). Ginseng has also been reported to stimulate testosterone secretion in male lab animals.

LH also stimulates the secretion of testosterone in men, and in the Jianxi studies, the testosterone increase was 45 percent to 90 percent.

Although both ginseng and deer antler have been used for a very long time in China to treat menstrual disorders and male impotence, such studies provide a clue about how they work. By modulating hormone production in the pituitary gland, the production of testosterone and other sex hormones in the adrenal gland, ovary, or testicle is affected.

Italian studies on ginseng suggest that it affects the adrenal glands by strongly stimulating the hypothalamus and pituitary gland.

More evidence is available that ginseng does something related to female cycles. A double-blind study conducted by the Institute for Traditional

Bright Idea
Read up on the herbs you're interested in, using a reputable herbal database, and check them out with your doctor as well. Appendixes B and C list some sources of herb information.

Medicine in Portland, Oregon, found that hefty doses of ginseng—on the order of 3 to 4.5 grams daily—appeared to influence women's menstrual cycles. Of the women who used ginseng for three weeks, 29 percent reported changes in the length of their cycles or their patterns of bleeding.

Table 13.1 lists the different ginsengs and describes their typical actions.

Note! ➜
The best and most potent ginsengs are said to come from the oldest roots (some are more than 30 years old) and from wild rather than cultivated plants.

TABLE 13.1: GINSENGS

Name	Also Called	Reputed Actions
American ginseng		A cool ginseng that is more appropriate for women than the warmer varieties. A deeply nourishing tonic for Yin and Qi. Somewhat moistening.
Korean ginseng	Red ginseng (heaven grade refers to the most potent yang variety)	The most warming and invigorating of the ginsengs. Used by athletes. Stimulates the endocrine system.
Shiu Chu ginseng		Means *first pick*. Highest grade of cultivated Chinese ginseng, produced from the oldest ginseng roots. Not as warming as Korean ginseng.
Siberian ginseng		Actually a cousin of the ginseng family. Well respected as an adaptogen, blood tonic, and adrenal tonic.
Chinese ginseng		A moderate-acting ginseng.
Panax pseudoginseng		A blood and cardiovascular tonic.

Prince ginseng	Radix pseudostellaria	Mild relative of the ginsengs. A Yin and Qi tonic. Has moistening properties. Protects against stress. Aids the digestive and respiratory systems.
Dong Quai	Tang Kuei	Not really a ginseng, but sometimes referred to as women's ginseng because of its widespread use as a blood tonic for regulating the menstrual cycle.

Ayurveda's Indian prescription

India's age-old holistic healing methods are known collectively as Ayurveda, a system of preserving well-being developed some 3,000 to 5,000 years ago. Like traditional Chinese medicine, Ayurveda focuses on the idea of balancing body energies.

According to Ayurveda, people usually exhibit a tendency toward one or more of three doshas, though everyone has some characteristics of each type. The doshas could be thought of as body, temperament and energy types—Vata, Pitta, or Kapha. Though two women may have the same ailment, treatment can differ if they're of different dosha makeup. A balance of all three doshas is considered healthful.

Vata

Vata comes from the Sanskrit vaayu ("that which moves") and so is associated with movement. In the body it corresponds to space and air. Balanced Vata contributes to creativity and change, but when imbalanced or overloaded it produces an anxious,

66

It is generally agreed by researchers today that ginseng exerts its effects on what is called the "pituitary, hypothalamus, adrenal axis." The term indicates the coordinated functions of these three glands in regulating metabolism, response, and homeostasis. Furthermore, this set of interacting glands may have been indirectly recognized for centuries by the Chinese as a functional unit influencing stress, aging, sexual function, and overall vitality.
—Subhuti Dharmananda, Ph.D., Director, Institute for Traditional Medicine, Portland, Oregon

99

high-strung nature. Someone who is Vata-dominant might likely be thin, active, and perceptive.

Vata people can find themselves susceptible to nervous system disorders and ailments having to do with the idea of air, such as respiratory illness, dry skin and joint problems. In general the characterics associated with Vata include: dry, cold, rough, subtle, light, fast, small, moving, and clear.

Pitta

In Ayurveda Pitta corresponds to the elements fire and water and rules the body's metabolism (including such functions as maintaining appropriate body temperature, digestion, and absorbing nutrients). Balanced Pitta is described as fostering the intellect, but when imbalanced leads to anger.

Generally the attributes associated with Pitta include: hot, sharp, acidic, and light. A Pitta-predominant individual would characteristically be of moderate girth and stature, ruddy-skinned, outspoken, and intelligent. Ailments Pitta people tend to be susceptible to have to do with their fiery nature—things like inflammation, fever, ulcers, and hypertension.

Kapha

The Kapha dosha is said to correspond to earth and water. The body's physical makeup comes from Kapha energy. It governs everything from bones and muscles to fluid circulation and immunity. Balanced Kapha suggests love and placidity but when imbalanced results in overattachment and greed.

A Kapha-dominant person may often be overweight, calm, and caring. Water diseases are the problem with this dosha—flus (and other ailments involving mucus), edema, weight gain, and slow metabolism are typical. The qualities associated with the Kapha dosha include: heavy, oily, cold, moist, dull, slow, and solid.

Ayurvedic balancing

How do you balance the doshas? Various ways, but the common sense idea of like increasing like is central to Ayurveda. If you are too cold already, eating or drinking cold things will only make you colder. To balance cold, eat more warm foods.

After a detailed analysis of your symptoms and dosha tendencies, an Ayurvedic practitioner can prescribe herbs, foods, activities, and certain Ayurvedic treatments to help balance your constitution. Excess Vata, for instance, might be countered by seeking an environment with less commotion, avoiding cold foods and taking steam baths—each of which has qualities opposite from Vata's characteristics. When eating to balance the doshas, consider the guidelines in Table 13.2.

TABLE 13.2: DOSHA-REGULATING FOODS

To Increase	To Decrease
Vata	pungent, bitter, astringent, sweet, salty, sour
Pitta	sour, salty, pungent sweet, astringent, bitter
Kapha	sweet, salty, sour, bitter, astringent, pungent

If you have mostly Vata characteristics, you can seek balance by:

- Following a Vata-pacifying diet
- Staying warm
- Taking on a gentle exercise routine
- Developing your abilities of caring and devotion
- Avoiding overstimulation and anxiety

If you're predominantly Pitta:

- Follow a Pitta-pacifying diet

- Seek cool surroundings
- Avoid overstimulation
- Develop your abilities to get along with people

And if you're Kapha, you can help balance that dosha by:

- Following a Kapha-pacifying diet
- Avoiding cold and wet
- Incorporating more movement and excitement into your life
- Developing your ability to give unselfishly

In Ayurveda, menopause can be seen as a transition in a woman's life from the active, outward Pitta to the philosophical state of Vata. Unbalanced Vata is held responsible for insomnia, thinning of vaginal tissue and skin, and nervous behavior. But the metabolism-regulating Pitta dosha is implicated in hot flashes and night sweating. Treatment concentrates on pacifying the Pitta and Vata doshas.

Ayurvedic herbs used in balancing the doshas are also known for their ability to treat specific ailments, and scientific studies have been done on many. A combination of tonic herbs is often used, with one or more key herbs known for specific properties.

Wild asparagus known in Sanskrit as Shatavari translates as "she who can satisfy a hundred husbands." It is among the major rejuvenating herbs taken by women following Ayurveda. Beyond its uses in menopause and as a general female tonic, the herb is used to stimulate libido and, in new mothers, milk secretion. It also has somewhat diuretic and calming qualities.

Excessive menstruation, hot flashes and PMS symptoms are often treated with Ashok (Saraca

Indica bark). Gotu kola is an Indian herb popularly available in the United States. It is traditionally used as a memory and intellect enhancer, as well as a blood purifier and builder in conditions such as anemia and amenorrhea. It is also used to treat skin conditions and is used in the treatment of hot flashes. Turmeric is also considered a blood purifier and blood builder.

Many different herbs are used in Ayurveda, and there is some crossover with those used in traditional Chinese medicine—Dong Quai, for instance, the extremely popular women's tonic herb. And turmeric is commonly used in Western cooking.

Other herbal traditions

China and India have not been the exclusive domain of herbal use. Throughout history, folklore, and literature, herbs have been intimately tied to daily life elsewhere in the world. Many mentions of herbs, interestingly, have to do with fertility—be it the mistletoe used in doorways at Christmas or the reference to the herbs "parsley, sage, rosemary, and thyme" in the old English folk song "Scarborough Fair." The herbs mentioned in Scarborough Fair are thought to have comprised a love potion, and the song itself is considered a riddle in which, perhaps, a girl's quick wit wins her a husband. And according to *A Dictionary of Plant-Lore* (by Roy Vickery, Oxford University Press, 1997), parsley, sage, and rosemary are said to grow best in households where the wife is the dominant member of the family. Parsley traditionally represented festivity, sage long life and wisdom, rosemary remembrance and thyme a hint of daring.

As to medicinal uses of the herbs mentioned, Nicholas Culpepper's 17th century tome *The English*

Timesaver
Ayurvedic herbs and combinations are available in many health food stores and by mail order, some specifically geared toward menopausal health.

Physician claims each will bring on the menstrual period. Sage has been suggested to aid conception. Rosemary baths were recommended before 1600 as an invigorating libido enhancer. And thyme was used to regulate the menstrual cycle and also during childbirth. However, many herbalists recommend avoiding all four herbs *during* pregnancy, due to their reputation as early abortifacients.

Today, certain herbs still have strong reputation for helping with specific problems, such as the following:

- *Hot flashes:* fennel, sage, ginseng, and dong quai

- *Water retention:* nettle, uva ursi, and chickweed

- *Estrogen replacement:* licorice, sarsaparilla, ginger, false unicorn root, black cohosh, red clover, and evening primrose oil

- *Progesterone support:* wild yam and chaste tree berry (vitex)

- *Anxiety and sleeplessness:* chamomile, valerian, kava kava, black cohosh, and passionflower

- *Mood swings:* chamomile, valerian, kava kava, black cohosh, passionflower, dandelion root, ginger, and St. John's wort

Bright Idea
Read up on the herbs you're interested in, using a reputable herbal database, and check them out with your doctor as well. Appendixes B and C lists some sources of herb information.

There is no doubt that some herbs are dangerous, and more than a few can evoke serious side effects if they're taken in a haphazard way—if too much is ingested, if they're taken in combination with certain other herbs or drugs, or if the wrong parts of a plant are used. People who are in delicate health to begin with should be especially cautious. A variety of herbs are reported to have toxic effects on the liver, for example, so anyone who has liver problems should tread carefully.

The negative effects of some herbs include problems with *ma huang* or *ephedra*. Ephedrine is used in over-the-counter nasal decongestants, with appropriate warnings and specified limitations on its use. As a food supplement, however, ephedra and its derivatives have been promoted for weight loss, energy, body-building, and other purposes.

Close to 20 deaths in the United States have been associated with the use of supplements that contain ephedrine alkaloids (a constituent of ephedra), and many adverse reactions have also been reported. Ephedrine is now prohibited in the sale of food supplements in Argentina because of adverse reactions and concerns that warnings were not being listed on packages.

The U.S. Food and Drug Administration has proposed a maximum allowable level of ephedrine alkaloids in dietary supplements. The FDA also proposes that labels state how long you should take a supplement that contains these compounds. Canada regulates products that contain ephedrine.

Watch Out!
The side effects of ephedra include dizziness, headaches, tremors, heart attack, and stroke. Always get a doctor's opinion before you try this powerful herb.

Beyond the herbal horizons

Two distinct types of alternative healing methods exist: those that involve taking something and those that rely on manipulation of the body's energy patterns.

Homeopathy fits into the former category. In the latter group are such established bodywork methods as acupuncture; various types of massage, such as shiatsu; and therapies that deal with energy flow, such as a form of Qi Gong.

Homeopathy for menopause

An 18th-century physician and pharmacist named Dr. Samuel Hahnemann began the classical practice of homeopathy, a branch of treatment whose name

Watch Out!
Strong-smelling substances such as camphor, coffee, and tea tree oil are thought to interfere with homeopathic healing, causing the original symptoms to return. The action is described as acting as an antidote to a homeopathic remedy (although the remedies themselves are not toxic). If you're going to try homeopathy, eschew the heavy scents.

derives from the Greek *homoion* (similar) and *pathos* (suffering). Homeopathic practice is governed by the law of similars. According to this philosophy, a medicine that can trigger a set of symptoms in a healthy person can cure the same symptoms.

Homeopathic remedies come from plant, mineral, and other sources. A small quantity is diluted, shaken, further diluted, and shaken again until a nearly infinitesimal amount of the original substance is left. Then the diluted substance is taken as a small pill (often, sublingually) or as drops. While the specific mechanisms by which homeopathy may actually work are unknown, the central idea behind it is that the body recognizes the minute quantity as an invader (in a way not unlike how vaccines work) and mounts its defenses to overcome the original problem. The greater the dilution (and the smaller the dose), the greater the reputed healing power.

Homeopathy has garnered some following in the United States; homeopathic remedies are widely available at health-food stores and some drugstores. But homeopathy is much more established in England, France, Switzerland, Germany, India, and other lands.

If you're interested in trying homeopathy, consult a practitioner or read up on the topic (see Appendix C for resources). Diagnosis can be complex and is based largely on observations about the type of person who can benefit from a given remedy. Also, homeopathic preparations may work best when you're not taking anything else that exerts a strong effect on your hormones.

There are two approaches to the administration of homeopathic remedies—the use of single remedies (which some homeopaths prefer) or the use of combination remedies geared for specific

Bright Idea
The Internet offers some good homeopathy resources. Try www.homeopathyhome.com for starters.

conditions (combination remedies are often named for the ailment they're used to treat). It's important to remember that homeopathic diagnosis takes into account not just the illness but also who is being treated and their characteristics. The person must fit the remedy as a whole.

Classic individual remedies that are sometimes used to treat menopausal symptoms include:

- Sepia (sometimes used for hot flashes)

- Pulsatilla (sometimes used for hot flashes)

- Sanguinaria

- Folliculinum

- Lachesis (sometimes used for hot flashes)

- Cimicifuga

- Salix nig.

- Zincum

- Thyroidinum

- Hypothalamus

- Aristolochia clematis (for cystitis)

- Natrum muriaticum (to regulate menstrual cycles)

- Luna

- Staphysagria

- Thuja

- Lac humanum (made from mother's milk)

Folliculinum, for example, is a homeopathic medicine made from synthetically produced estrone (an estrogen). Although the use of folliculinum is debated in traditional homeopathy, some practitioners report good results in using it to reduce PMS and to alleviate some problems in

Bright Idea
You can find a homeopath through the National Center for Homeopathy, 801 N. Fairfax St., Suite 306, Alexandria, VA, 22314, (703) 548-7790.

menopause—essentially, to help regulate hormonal control.

Some popular homeopathic remedies used for menopausal and menstrual difficulties are called by obvious names, such as hormonal comp (used to balance female hormones), "Menopause" or climacteric comp (used for menopausal symptoms), and female support (also used for hormone regulation). These are helpful names for preparations that contain one or more single remedies. In the remedy female support, for example, the medically active component is oophorinum sarcode, which is made from the ovary.

Acupuncture, massage, and energy work

Acupuncture is an age-old Asian healing method that relies on the concept of *energy meridians*, or channels, that run throughout the body. Western medicine is just beginning to address this concept. In acupuncture, minute needles are placed at key points in the meridians to affect the *Qi* (energy) and encourage its proper flow.

Many women find relief from hormonal problems via acupuncture, which generally involves a thorough consultation about the nature of your complaints and other aspects of your health. The practitioner may ask to see your tongue and will check your pulse in slightly different spots. The needles (which should be the single-use, disposable kind) are gently tapped in just below the skin at a few key points while you are reclining on a bed or table. The needles usually can barely be felt or cause minimal discomfort; they are very small. After about half an hour, the practitioner removes the needles.

The National Institutes of Health now recognizes acupuncture as providing successful treatment

Unofficially... Acupuncture is said to target a few specific points, whereas shiatsu covers many.

for a variety of conditions. Although the practice is less familiar than Western medicine, acupuncture has been shown to have similar success in treating some ailments, and many women report that it helps them with menopausal problems. Among other things, acupuncture has been shown in research to trigger endorphin release and thereby alleviate pain. Other research suggests that it has the capability to affect hormonal and neurotransmitter functions.

An alternative to acupuncture that does not involve needles is *acupressure,* which involves pressing on the same meridian points that acupuncture stimulates with needles. In *shiatsu,* an Asian form of pressure-point massage, you get the comforts of a rubdown with specific emphasis on many points that are otherwise accessed through acupuncture. A practitioner will query you about your health concerns before deciding on an appropriate pattern of massage. Shiatsu is very much a form of medical treatment, although it may be more enjoyable as a form of massage.

Among the other bodywork approaches to balance is a form of Qi Gong. Part of Qi Gong practice is an exercise, but another part of the practice involves the manipulation of a patient's energy by a Qi Gong practitioner, who uses his or her own energy in healing. This external healing is called external Qi Kung or Chi Sao, and it doesn't necessarily involve touching the patient. Rather, the practitioner uses his or her energy to redirect blocked energy in the patient's body into its proper flow.

Whether you're skeptical, intrigued, or a little of both, exploring alternative therapies at your own pace (and with a good deal of research) may net you benefits. Scams and charlatans abound in the realm of alternative medicine, but the mysterious ways that some treatments work may not be so mysterious in 10, 15, or 20 years, as conventional science investigates and seeks to understand them. Herbs, for example, are no longer in the realm of folk medicine. Scientific bases for the actions of herbs are being discovered, and herbs are undergoing some of the same double-blind tests that are used to test conventional medicines.

Just the facts

- Many herbs that are estrogenic also have antiestrogenic properties.

- Traditional Chinese medicine, which involves herbal therapy and acupuncture, has a long history in treating gynecologic and endocrinologic conditions.

- Acupuncture has been found to be effective for certain conditions, due to its capability to stimulate endorphin release and affect neurotransmitters.

- Fennel, sage, ginseng, and dong quai are among the herbs that have a reputation for helping hot flashes.

- Read up on herbs you're considering using and be careful with them—just because something is natural doesn't mean it can't hurt.

Estrogens from Everywhere

Chapter 14

Hormones don't only develop naturally in our bodies and come in a little pill that we can take for HRT at menopause. Many of the things that we eat every day contain hormones themselves, or at the least substances that can influence our body's own endocrine output. *Phytohormones* is the name given to the hormones produced by plants.

Xenohormones, however, include those hormone-influencing substances from some pesticides, plastics, and other chemicals that exert potentially dangerous hormonal actions in the environment, causing increasing worry among environmentalists.

In addition, hormones are given to livestock to enhance their growth. Hormone use in livestock means more meat and milk, and although studies attest to the safety of the practice, not everyone is convinced that humans won't feel the effects.

This chapter discusses the new popularity of phytohormones and tells you what foods may help your own hormonal status. The chapter also briefs you on the debate about hormone supplementation in farm animals and on the potential threat posed by unintended xenohormones in the environment.

Phytohormones: you are what you eat

Hormones occur in plants, sometimes at high concentrations, and a popular topic these days is the benefit of phytoestrogens to women, particularly to those who are coping with perimenopause and menopause. Phytoestrogens and other phytohormones are among the many naturally occurring chemicals in plants. Although these substances are not vitamins or minerals, they do exert actions and can have an influence in the plant, the lab, or the body, as many studies show.

There are several reasons for this interest in phytoestrogens and other phytosterols:

1. Despite multiple benefits of estrogen, only one in four menopausal women actually use HRT. The inconvenience of potential bleeding and concern over possible malignancy deter many women from taking conventional HRT.

2. In addition, there is a growing trend in the use of complementary and alternative medicine, with roughly one in three Americans using these therapies.

3. Many women armed with new sources of information not available even a decade ago are scouting out solutions to their quest for estrogen benefits with a more holistic approach.

Plants contain molecules that have a steroidal nucleus and therefore are known as *phytosterols*.

Some of these plant chemicals are similar or even indentical to a variety of our own steroid hormones and can exert similar effects in our systems, mimicking the steroid hormones that we produce, such as estrogen and progesterone. Although phytosterols have similar or identical structure to human hormone, when taken orally, they do not have hormonal activity until they are metabolized (broken down) in the liver, and so there can be variation in phytosterol activity from one individual to another depending on one's metabolism.

Phytohormones that have estrogenic activity are called phytoestrogens. There are several groups of phytoestrogens; the most important are called isoflavones and lignans. Foods that are high in isoflavones include soybeans, clover, chickpeas, and legumes. Lignans are found in whole cereals, flaxseed, bran, and legumes.

Phytohormones that have structures similar to progesterone belong to a group called sapogenins. Unlike phytoestrogens, sapogenins cannot be metabolized to an active form by the body. The body lacks the necessary enzymes. Sapogenins can only be converted into active progesterone in the lab.

Investigation of the effect of phytosterols (popularly called *phytohormones*) in humans has gained popularity relatively recently. Not everything is known about what phytosterols do in the body or how they do it. Knowledge of their side effects and potential drug interactions is also limited.

Interestingly, some of the plants that are now being found to have significant sterol quantities and hormonal effects in humans are the same plants that have been used in folk medicine for ages (cramp bark, for example).

Unofficially... Not every plant that exerts a hormonal effect actually contains specific mimicking sterols. Different plant substances can affect our hormones in other ways.

Many varieties of phytohormones exist, including isoflavones, lignans, and sapogenins.

A phytoestrogen primer

Asian women seem to sail through their menopause years with relatively minimal problems in comparison with Western women. But researchers have found that when Asian women give up their traditional diet and assume typical American eating habits, their advantage begins to disappear.

That finding has generated enthusiasm about soy. Soybeans, which are a staple in a wide variety of Asian fare, from tofu to miso and soy sauce, contain ingredients that have significant phytoestrogenic properties. Consequently, researchers suggest that soy is a major reason why Asian women fare well during menopause.

Here are some good sources of phytoestrogens:

- Soybeans and other legumes
- Other vegetables
- Fruits
- Whole grains and some seeds (such as flax)
- Certain herbs

Timesaver
You can find information about soy almost anywhere, including health-food stores and the Internet. You can investigate the benefits of soy products at the Soy and Human Health Web home page (www.ag.uiuc. edu/~stratsoy/ soyhealth/).

(See Chapter 13 for herbs that support estrogen activity in the body.)

Phytoestrogens are being credited with potential benefits such as easing the menopausal transition, ensuring bone and cardiovascular health, and reducing the risk of certain cancers. Recent studies suggest that when a woman's diet is high in phytoestrogens, her risk of breast cancer decreases. In one Australian study, women who had high levels of two byproducts of phytoestrogens (enterolactone and equol) in their urine had a lower breast-cancer risk than other women.

Despite the current rage for phytoestrogens and their apparently great benefits, keep the situation in perspective. Science doesn't provide definitive answers for every women's situation. In other studies on phytoestrogens, reduction in breast-cancer risk seemed to hold true for *pre*menopausal women who had high phytoestrogen intake, but not for *post*menopausal women.

How phytoestrogens work

Because estrogens are associated with cancer risk in some cases, it may seem odd that phytoestrogens have been found to potentially prevent breast cancer. That dilemma is the key to how phytoestrogens work.

Our own bodies produce certain estrogens that have strong actions in the body and others that are relatively weak in comparison. Though some phytoestrogens are quite potent, most tend to be weak estrogens and may actually act both in an estrogenic manner and also in an antiestrogenic way in the body, attaching to receptor sites that otherwise might be occupied by human estrogen, which would exert stronger, possibly unfavorable effects. It's hypothesized that phytoestrogens decrease breast cancer risk by binding to estrogen receptors in the breast, thus blocking stronger estrogens such as estradiol from activating these sites.

Soy for your hormones

Although plenty of foods contain phytoestrogens, you may hear the most about soy. Soy offers many nutritional benefits. It contains antioxidants (such as vitamin E and coenzyme Q-10) and can cut cholesterol. According to a 1995 study published in the *New England Journal of Medicine,* eating close to 2

Bright Idea
If you're on HRT and want to try regular use of phytoestrogen foods, talk to your doctor. Intake of additional phytoestrogens could affect your hormone prescription and results.

Watch Out!
Women vary in their reactions to phytoestrogens, as they do to other estrogens. If you're going to add phytoestrogens to your diet, start slowly. Some women report symptoms of excess estrogen (such as breast soreness) after a single glass of soy milk.

ounces of soy protein daily may reduce blood cholesterol by 10 percent in a month.

Soy can also be used to help with perimenopause and menopause. Soy is one of the sources from which estradiol and other estrogens can be manufactured in a lab, and it's a rich source of phytoestrogens outside the lab.

Soy contains *isoflavones,* which are weak phytoestrogens made up of molecules similar to the estrogen molecules that our bodies make. *Genistein,* the most widely touted soy isoflavone, is available in capsules and tablets as a dietary supplement. *Daidzein* is another important isoflavone that occurs in soy.

The following soy foods are all high in isoflavones, offering 30 to 50 milligrams per serving:

- (roasted) Soy nuts (1 ounce)
- Soy flour (½ cup)
- Soy grits (¼ cup)
- Textured soy protein (½ cup, cooked)
- Yellow vegetable, green vegetable, or black soybeans (½ cup, cooked)
- Soy milk (1 cup)
- Tempeh (½ cup)
- Tofu (½ cup)

Unofficially...
Women who need estrogen therapy but who are at risk of breast cancer are often prescribed estrogen manufactured from soy.

Soy isoflavones may help counter some menopause problems, but not others. In an Italian study, postmenopausal women used 60 grams daily of protein powder that was either composed mainly of the milk protein casein or of soy protein (similar to about two servings of a soy-rich food). Over the course of 12 weeks, the incidence of hot flashes fell in both groups—by 45 percent in the women who ate soy, but by just 30 percent in both the placebo group and the group that used milk-based protein. Other symptoms—such as headaches, depression, and insomnia—weren't affected by soy, but other studies suggest that soy isoflavones may reduce sweating and insomnia.

A short course in estrogen-receptor science may explain these results. For years, scientists knew about only one type of estrogen receptor, which was dubbed ER alpha. But another type—ER beta—has been discovered. ER beta receptors are found largely in bone, bladder tissues, and the cardiovascular system. Genistein, an abundant soy isoflavone, binds weakly to ER alpha receptors, but nearly as well as estrogen itself to ER beta receptors.

Researchers suggest that this phenomenon explains why soy plays an important role in preserving bone health and may account for lower rates of heart disease in countries where soy is served regularly. Soy isoflavones may be beneficial for the following conditions:

- Typical menopausal symptoms (hot flashes, insomnia, vaginal dryness, night sweats, etc.)
- Cardiovascular health
- Bone density
- Risk of uterine or breast cancers

Soy isoflavones do not appear to have beneficial effects on the brain. Studies do not show improvement in memory or cognition the way traditionally prescribed estrogen does. Similarly, there is no effect on the vagina or bladder. Women with urogenital atrophy will not get relief of vaginal dryness with isoflavones.

If you want to try adding more soy to your diet, a trip to a natural-foods supermarket or a good

Unofficially...
The right amount of soy isoflavones varies for each woman. Asians eat about 20 to 80 milligrams daily, whereas average American intake is more like 1 to 3 milligrams per day.

health-food store should give you plenty of options. You can also find soy products at regular grocery stores. Check the Asian-foods section for some varieties, the produce or dairy section for tofu, and the dairy or diet section for soy milk. Even frozen tofu and soy-milk desserts, similar to ice cream, are available.

Beyond soy: Other phytoestrogen foods

Watch Out!
Soy oil typically does not contain isoflavones, but it has other health benefits. If you're supplementing for phytoestrogens, choose another source.

Soy is only one of many foods that are stocked with phytoestrogens. You can also find phytoestrogens in legumes such as lentils and in garbanzo, kidney, lima, and black beans. Other sources include whole grains (oats, corn, rice, millet, and buckwheat) and some fruits, vegetables, and herbs, such as rhubarb, carrots, and sage.

Diosgenin and B-sitosterol are two common plant steroids that can have an estrogenic action. The former substance occurs in a wide range of wild-yam species. Wild yams are used to manufacture hormones (estrogen, progesterone, and progestins) for human use. Although wild-yam creams are popular among women who are seeking a source of natural progesterone (which actually needs to be lab-synthesized), diosgenin can have phytoestrogenic effects. So can B-sitosterol (a component of soy), saw palmetto, and red clover, as you see in Chapter 13.

We mentioned that certain plants contain hormones identical to human hormones. Table 14.1 lists some of those common botanicals. However, bear in mind that the estrogens are only in trace amounts for some of these, and they do not necessarily occur in the edible portion.

TABLE 14.1: HUMAN HORMONES IN THE PLANT WORLD

Plants with Estrone	Plants with Estriol	Plants with Estradiol
Pomegranates	Licorice	Hops
Apples	Green beans	Pomegranates
Corn		
Hops		
Olives		

Source: Botanical Medicines Acting on the Female Reproductive System, Jill Stansbury, M.D.

Increasing the proportion of natural foods that you eat is a great policy for your health and could affect how easily you get through menopause. Natural foods have important health benefits that stretch way beyond their phytohormone content.

Hormones in the meat you eat

The surge in the use of organically grown food—vegetables, fruits, and grains—isn't limited to the plant kingdom. Organic meats are also attracting interest among consumers who are concerned about food additives. Some of those concerns involve hormonal supplementation of livestock and its potential effect in the human body.

A bountiful, tasty meat supply at an economical production cost is a chief goal of livestock farmers. Breeds are hybridized and the type of feed is selected to encourage meat production, just as a wheat farmer seeks to encourage the wheat harvest.

But another way to boost meat supply or milk production is to give cattle hormone supple-ments. Gonadotropins may be injected to stimulate ovulation and encourage reproduc-tion. Lab-manufactured growth hormone may be

Timesaver
Links to recipes, health informa-tion, and other information about soy are available on the Internet. Try the U.S. Soyfoods Directory, main-tained by the Indiana Soybean Board, at www.soyfoods. com.

Unofficially...
Canada's federal health department has decided *not* to approve the bovine growth hormone reST for use in that country. One committee studying it found no ill effects in humans, but Canada rejected the hormone after a panel of veterinarians concluded it poses an unacceptable risk to the health of cattle.

administered to stimulate milk production. Estrogen may be used to enhance meat quantity.

The use of supplemental bovine growth hormone (BGH), to stimulate milk production in cows has generated considerable controversy, even though the U.S. Food and Drug Administration approved its use during the mid-1990s. Critics are concerned about not only potential long-term effects in cows and in consumers, but also the possibility of increased frequency of breast infections (and, thus, increased use of antibiotics) in cows receiving BGH.

The FDA and other health organizations have concluded that both milk and meat from BGH-supplemented cows are safe for human consumption; however, some health advocates remain unconvinced. Among their concerns is the presence of a second growth hormone (insulinlike growth factor-I, or IGF-I) in milk from BGH-supplemented cows. Some industry studies showed an increase of IGF-I from 25 percent to 70 percent, and a 1989 study found increases of IGF-I at least 3.6 times higher in cows treated with BGH for one week compared with untreated cows.

This growth factor occurs naturally in human saliva and breast milk, but in trace quantities. Too much of it can cause acromegaly (giantism), blood-sugar disorders, and blood-pressure abnormalities, and its potential role in certain cancers (including breast cancer) is still unknown. According to a review by the Congressional Office of Technology Assessment in the early '90s, however, taking IGF-1 with your glass of milk has no effect:

> Similar to results with bST (BGH), studies with laboratory animal models have demonstrated that IGF-1 has no biological activity if

administered orally. The importance of increased amounts of IGF-I in milk from bST-treated animals is uncertain. However, the amount of IGF-I ingested in 1 liter of milk approximates the amount of IGF-I in saliva swallowed daily by adults.

Unwanted estrogens in the environment

Can the air we breathe, the water we drink, and the things we touch really play havoc with our hormones? Yes. Just ask the U.S. Environmental Protection Agency.

The EPA has been concerned for some time about chemicals that can interfere with our endocrine systems. These chemicals, called *endocrine disruptors*, include strong synthetic estrogens that may play a role in declining sperm counts in human males and in deformed genitalia, unusual mating behaviors, and sterility in animal populations.

These xenoestrogens are present in many substances, such as some pesticides and some plastics. Because they're not easily broken down, xenoestrogens may find their way into waterways and remain there.

Some chemicals mimic natural hormones, and the body responds; others block the effects of our own hormones; and still others stimulate or inhibit the production of our hormones. Endocrine disruptors can cause problems in the following ways:

- Mimicking our hormones, thereby oversupplying their effect

- Blocking receptor sites, thereby preventing hormone action

- Stimulating the growth of more hormone receptors, thereby heightening the effects of our hormones and xenohormones

- Changing our hormones, thereby altering hormone expression or growth

- Depleting hormones by accelerating their reuptake

- Inhibiting reuptake of hormones, thereby causing a lingering effect

One endocrine disruptor may work synergistically with another to compound the effect, or a veritable soup of chemicals may be at work.

Pollutants and pesticides

Just as estrogen is largely responsible for the development of breasts and a feminine shape in human girls at puberty, estrogen can have a feminizing effect in males—not only humans, but animals as well. Xenoestrogens in the environment are suspected of being responsible for this effect.

The pesticide DDT, which was banned from use in the United States in 1972, was found to have estrogenic properties. DDT was implicated in the thinning of bird eggshells, the development of female gonads in male offspring, and even changes in parenting behavior.

The saga of Lake Apopka in Central Florida illustrates the potentially devastating effects of endocrine disruptors. Scientists at the University of Florida believe a large pesticide spill along the shores of that already polluted lake is implicated in reduced rates of alligator reproduction and survival, with increased numbers of females being born in comparison to healthy males.

The chemical DDE, a DDT breakdown product which is believed to be largely responsible for the situation at Lake Apopka, binds to androgen (male hormone) receptors and blocks them in as small a quantity as 60 parts per billion. Concentrations as high as 3,570 parts per billion were found in stillborn human infants in Atlanta during the mid-1960s. Quantities of 5,800 parts per billion were isolated in affected alligator eggs, and among workers in countries where the pesticide is still used, levels as high as 140 parts per billion have been identified.

The decline in the population of wild Florida panthers was once attributed to poaching, but experts now worry that feminization due to estrogens in the environment decreased sperm count in male panthers, thereby leading to the decline. Pesticides and herbicides are now banned in national parks in the Southeast.

Scientists are concerned not only about animal populations, but also about us. The rates of certain reproductive cancers have increased over the past 50 years. Testicular-cancer incidence has tripled, for example. During the same period, fertility rates have decreased, due in part to declining sperm counts.

Endocrine disruptors are not unique to the United States; virtually every industrialized country faces the same problems. In Great Britain, for example, pollution watchdogs warn that a high proportion of the male fish in nearly all of Britain's rivers are carrying eggs—an obviously female trait. Feminization and gender-bending effects are characteristic of xenoestrogenic contamination.

Research initiatives totaling millions of U.S. dollars were launched into the issue of endocrine disruptors in Britain in 1998. Announcing the projects, British Environment Minister Michael Meacher explained, "We are all aware of reports of declining sperm counts and quality, increases in testicular

Unofficially...
Male fertility is down. In 1940, sperm density was estimated at 113 million per millimeter of semen, but by 1990, the density was reduced to about 66 million—a 20 percent decline.

Watch Out!
Some women are very sensitive even to phyto-estrogens. Don't assume that a plant-based estrogen is necessarily a weak estrogen.

cancer in men, birth defects in baby boys and reports of effects in wildlife, particularly fish."

When dealing with questions about the potential harm in our environment, scientists are trying to balance healthy inquiry and healthy skepticism. Some disturbing questions have yet to be answered.

Environmentalists point out that physicians have theories that explain only about a third of all the breast cancer that occurs. Genetic predisposition may account for about 5 percent. Other factors may increase risk, such as early onset of menstruation, late menopause, not having children, and not having breast-fed. Too much estrogen and radiation also contribute to breast-cancer risk. But there are no readily identifiable causes for the majority of breast-cancer cases.

Some studies have found links between certain pesticides and breast cancer, and the possibility remains that man-made factors in the environment, such as xenohormones, may contribute to the risk. Some xenohormones exert their effects mainly at certain stages in human development: before birth, during infancy, and during puberty. The link among these times is a high growth rate because the body is using hormones to perform particularly ambitious tasks.

Environmentally available estrogens

Certain plants can exhibit pronounced estrogenic activity, and some of our own hormones exert pronounced activity, but neither type of hormone is in the same league as the man-made materials that may be leaching synthetic estrogens into the environment. A nearly infinitesimal quantity of some synthetic xenoestrogens has a potent effect.

Plant hormones can act as endocrine disruptors, but their effects aren't likely to be long-lived unless daily exposure occurs. Naturally occurring estrogens in plants are soluble in water and dissipate easily. Chemicals that have come into use during this century, however, tend to be stable substances that are capable of building up in fat and other tissues, and that are not easily eradicated. In addition, proteins in the human body that work to eliminate excess hormone levels may not recognize some synthetic estrogens.

The great unknown

No one has a catalog of every endocrine disruptor that has come into our ecosystem since the Industrial Revolution, so many unknowns exist. Environmental toxicologists are just beginning to put together a picture of how serious the health threat may be. The U.S. government has already banned the use of some chemicals that have raised concern about possible endocrine-disrupting effects, including PCBs, and the pesticides DDT, chlordane, aldrin/dieldrin, endrin, heptachlor, kepone, toxaphene, and 2,4,5-T.

Along with some pesticides, some plastics and substances used in plastic production are suspected of exerting hormonal activity, and the list goes on to include byproducts of other industries and pollutants.

Another type of chemical, phthalates, helps make some plastics flexible, and certain heavy metals are widely used in the production of plastics. The potential for chemical leaching from some plastics is particularly worrisome when the plastic may be used for food storage.

Unofficially...
More testing is being done in an attempt to ensure the safety of plastics and plasticizers. The minute quantities of hormonally active substances that can cause endocrine disruption, however, make identifying these substances much more difficult than searching for the proverbial needle in a haystack.

Watch Out!
DDT is still used
outside the
United States,
including many
developing
countries.

In the mid-1990s, the Food Quality Protection Act and Safe Drinking Water Act mandated the EPA to come up with a screening and testing strategy for endocrine disruptors, to be implemented before 2000. New pesticides and other chemicals are routinely screened for potential endocrine effects, and scientists are also screening chemicals that have been used for many years.

Scientists want to know more about the classes of chemicals that may affect the endocrine system, how much it takes to induce effects, and how humans and animals are exposed to the chemicals (by ingestion, inhalation, or touch). A big question is what happens when a person is exposed to multiple chemicals. Endocrine-disruption effects may be additive.

A committee formed by the EPA to look into such questions recommended the screening of six types of mixtures:

- Contaminants in human breast milk
- Phytoestrogens in soy-based infant formula
- Mixtures of chemicals commonly found at hazardous waste sites
- Pesticide/fertilizer mixtures
- Disinfection byproducts
- Gasoline

Since androgens, estrogens, and thyroid hormone are such key controls in the body, the committee also recommended testing for endocrine disruption of all three.

Keeping healthy

To keep healthy, keep informed about matters that pertain to your health. Scan articles in your local paper and in magazines, check the EPA's endocrine-disruptor information site on the Internet (www.epa.gov/opptintr/opptendo), or check with an environmental group in your community.

If you are particularly worried about potential endocrine disruptors in your environment, you can take the following steps to reduce contact with them:

- Emphasize fresh, organically grown food in your diet. What about non-organic foods? The EPA does not think that consumers need to switch to organic food based on dietary risk concerns, and notes, as pointed out by the NAS and others, pesticide residues in food are generally present at low levels unlikely to present significant risks.

- Thoroughly rinse your fruits and vegetables in water, scrub them, and peeling when necessary. Cooking reduces some pesticide residues further, according to the EPA.

- Don't microwave food in plastics not designed for such use, and generally keep foods that come in plastics away from excess heat.

- As much as possible, use soaps, cleaners, cosmetics, and other preparations that originate from natural products, rather than those that contain a complex blend of chemicals.

- Avoid obvious sources of pollution.

- Rely on nonchemical pesticides for your home or garden.

- Drink spring water (packaged in glass bottles if you like). What about *tap water*? The EPA regulates certain chemicals suspected of being endocrine disruptors in drinking water, and

Unofficially... According to the U.S. Environmental Protection Agency, most fish that is sold in supermarkets and restaurants comes from the ocean and is much less likely to have detectable levels of PCBs and DDT/DDE than freshwater fish are.

Timesaver
The FDA has a wealth of information about cosmetics and toiletries at its Internet site: http://www.fda.gov.

says most regulatory levels are protective for the individual chemicals but uncertainty remains in specific cases and for the cumulative effect of multiple exposures. The EPA believes a public water supply that meets Federal drinking water standards provides safe drinking water. What about *plastic bottles?* The EPA says there is currently no indication contaminant leaching (nor the water source) is a problem in bottled water, and thus that bottled water is generally safe to drink.

■ If you have a private well, consider having its water tested (since the Safe Drinking Water Act doesn't regulate private wells). The EPA advises that private well owners who suspect a potential for contamination have the water tested—such as in the case of a shallow well in an agricultural area with heavy pesticide use. You can ask the assistance of your appropriate state authority in testing your private well water (at a certified lab) for the same potential endocrine disruptors that are regulated in public drinking water.

■ The EPA notes that if you fish, you can check with state authorities to ensure the freshwater areas you frequent are safe from environmental hazards.

■ Some chemical residues concentrate in fatty tissue. If you're very concerned about limiting your exposure to them, opting for lean cuts is one option.

However unsettling the fact may be, the average person's largest source of exposure to xenoestrogens and other endocrine disruptors may be from their own body burden of chemicals, according to the World Wildlife Fund, Canada. On average, environmental scientists say, humans have at least 250 chemical contaminants in their body fat, regardless of where they live.

Giving your body a regular daily intake of mildly acting phytoestrogens may displace xenoestrogens that could otherwise gain access to estrogen receptors. Scientific testing to support this theory remains to be done, however. There's no shortage of chemicals and potential problems—just a shortage of time in which to test the myriad combinations that may produce endocrine effects.

Just the facts

- Many legumes, vegetables, fruits, and herbs have phytohormone activity in the body.

- Soy is a rich source of phytoestrogens that may help prevent disease.

- Although the U.S. Food and Drug Administration says that the use of hormones in livestock is safe, some health advocates remain worried about the long-term effects on humans.

- Hormone disruptors are increasingly being found in the environment.

Bright Idea
Natural-foods grocery stores often carry environmentally friendly cleaning supplies. You can also find simple products at your regular supermarket that can be used in a variety of ways. You can use baking soda, for example, to brush your teeth or to scrub your sink.

Glossary

acupuncture Traditional Chinese medical practice of treating illness through the placing of small needles in the skin at strategic energy points.

adaptogen A substance (herb, pharmaceutical, or food) reputed to enhance balance and help the body better adjust to changes and resist disease.

adrenaline Epinephrine; a stress hormone that is secreted from the adrenal medulla which plays a role in "fight or flight" responses.

alendronate Anti-resorptive medication for use by women past menopause; the first nonhormonal therapy on the market for osteoporosis. By inhibiting the breakdown of skeletal bone by osteoclasts, alendronate (which is thus a bisphosphonate) can not only cut down on the loss of bone but also allow its mass to increase.

Alzheimer's disease Degenerative disease of the central nervous system characterized by senility; named for the German physician Alois Alzheimer.

amenorrhea The abnormal absence of regular monthly menstruation.

androgen Any of a number of masculinizing hormones present in the male or female body.

androstenediol An androgenic (masculinizing) hormone made in the ovaries and adrenals that can be metabolized in fatty tissues into the estrogens estradiol and estrone (or can be converted to testosterone). After menopause, it supports estrogen levels by increased conversion to estrone in fat, muscle, and other tissues.

androstenedione An androgenic (masculinizing) hormone present in male and female bodies that can be converted into estrogens or testosterone.

andropause Gradual changes that take place in men as their sex-hormone production declines; the male alternative to the female menopause.

anovulatory Not ovulating; a menstrual cycle characterized by lack of ovulation.

BGH (bovine growth hormone) Bovine somatotrophin or BST; a hormone used to boost milk and meat production in livestock.

cervical mucus Mucus detectable in the vagina that changes throughout the menstrual cycle. Its qualities can be an indicator of ovulation.

cervix The narrow outer end of the uterus that protrudes into the vagina.

change, the Menopause.

cholesterol The precursor to steroid hormones and sex hormones in the body.

circadian rhythm The cycles of the body that occur in a 24-hour or almost 24-hour rhythm; affected by lengths of light and dark periods, among other things.

climacteric Menopause; also used to define the several years leading up to menopause and following it when hormonal changes are noticed.

colorectal cancer   Cancer of the colon and/or rectum; the second most diagnosed cancer and second-most cause of death by cancer in the United States.

corpus luteum   Literally *yellow body;* a yellow-colored and progesterone-secreting tissue mass that forms after ovulation from the ovarian follicle after it has released an egg.

designer hormones   Hormone or hormonelike pharmaceuticals that target specific actions in the body but avoid others.

diosgenin   A by-product formed in the processing of plants from which certain steroid hormones are synthesized, such as progesterone synthesized from wild yam.

dysmenorrhea   Painful menstruation (such as with cramping).

endocrine   Refers to ductless glands (such as the thyroid and pituitary) or tissue that produces secretions that are carried in the bloodstream.

endocrine disruptors   Chemicals that can interfere with the functioning of human or animal endocrine systems, such as causing abnormal mating behavior or sterility.

endometrial hyperplasia   Overgrowth of the uterine lining; may require treatment using progestins; seen with menstrual irregularities during peri-menopause and menopause.

endometriosis   The growth of uterine lining tissue in other pelvic areas.

endometrium   The nutrient-rich mucous membrane lining of the uterus.

ERT (estrogen replacement therapy)   The replacement of estrogen by an outside source when depleted in the body. The term HRT (hormone replacement therapy) may also be used to refer to estrogen replacement therapy.

estradiol   Also known as E2; the main human estrogen (a "strong" estrogen) produced in the ovaries.

estriol   Also known as E3; an estrogen that is a relatively weak metabolite of estradiol; produced in larger quantities in the body during pregnancy.

estrogen, or estrogens   The name for a group of substances that have feminizing effects in the body; sex hormones that promote estrus and stimulate female secondary sex characteristics (such as breast development in puberty).

estrone   Also known as E1; a weak estrogen made largely from estradiol. After menopause it is the main estrogen produced in the female body, largely through conversion of androgens in fatty and other tissues.

fertility   In women, the ability to become pregnant via periodic ovulation; more generally, having the capability to produce offspring.

fibroids   Areas of fibrous growth in the uterus (benign tumors).

follicle   Also called graafian follicle; the moist cavity in an ovary that contains a mature egg before ovulation.

follicular phase   That early phase of the menstrual cycle following menstruation when follicles are growing in the ovary, prior to ovulation; also described as the proliferative phase.

FSH (follicle-stimulating hormone)   Hormone secreted by the anterior pituitary gland that stimulates development of the ovarian follicles and the production of estrogen. FSH is a gonadotropic hormone.

genistein   A well-known soy isoflavone (weak estrogen).

GnRH (gonadotropin-releasing hormone) A hormone sent by the hypothalamus gland to the pituitary, prompting the release of either FSH (follicle-stimulating hormone) or LH (luteinizing hormone).

gonad Reproductive glands (the ovaries or testis).

gonadotropic That which stimulates the gonads, as in gonadotropic hormones.

homeopathy An alternative medical system that treats ailments by giving minute, many-times-diluted doses of a remedy that would, in healthy persons, produce symptoms like those of the disease.

hormone A substance produced by cells that circulates in body fluids and exerts specific effects on cells elsewhere in the body.

hot flash A very typical type of discomfort seen in menopause and perimenopause, characterized by a sudden brief flushing and feeling of heat; caused by rapid dilation of capillaries and associated with hormonal imbalance.

hot flush See **hot flash.**

HRT (hormone replacement therapy) The replacement by an outside source of one or more hormones depleted in the body; in menopause, refers largely to dual estrogen and progesterone replacement—ERT is estrogen replacement therapy, though the term may be used to refer to any hormone replaced in connection with menopause.

hysterectomy Subtotal hysterectomy: removal of the uterus only; total hysterectomy: removal of the uterus and cervix; total hysterectomy with bilateral oophorectomy: removal of the uterus, cervix, and both ovaries.

infertility In a woman, inability to conceive (or sustain) a pregnancy due to any number of factors;

usually refers to inability to conceive prior to normal menopause.

isoflavone Weak phytoestrogen similar to the estrogen molecules our bodies make. Genistein is a major soy isoflavone.

LH (luteinizing hormone) A gonadotropic hormone secreted by the anterior pituitary gland that prompts ovulation.

luteal phase That late phase of the menstrual cycle following ovulation when the corpus luteum is secreting progesterone; also called the secretory phase in description of the condition of the uterine glands at that time.

mammography An X-ray or other scan of the breast; used to detect cancer and other abnormalities.

menarche The first menstrual period experienced in adolescence.

menopause The normal cessation of the menstrual cycle in women, occurring usually in their 40s or 50s; clinically defined when a woman has not had a period for a year; casually used to describe the period of time surrounding cessation of the menstrual cycle.

menstrual cycle Usually 28 days long (give or take a few); the first day of menstrual bleeding defines day 1 of each cycle; menstrual cycle refers to the changes that take place in a woman's body over this nearly month-long time span (to prepare for the possibility of pregnancy, and in the event there is no pregnancy, to shed the uterine lining and prepare again for fertility during the next cycle).

mittleschmertz A German term referring to pains that may be experienced around the time of ovulation.

noradrenaline Norepinephrine; precursor of the hormone epinephrine.

oophorectomy Surgical removal of one or both ovaries.

osteoporosis A condition of "brittle bones" that older women are at risk of developing. It is characterized by reduction in bone density and mass, and an increase in porosity. Osteoporosis leads to a higher risk of fractures. Estrogen and calcium have been found helpful in preventing osteoporosis development.

ovarian cysts Cysts in the ovaries arising from hormonal disruption and associated with irregular periods.

ovaries The pair of female reproductive organs on either side of your pelvis that produces eggs (and that secrete sex hormones).

ovulation The release of an egg from the ovarian follicle on or about day 14 of a woman's menstrual cycle; the height of a woman's fertility during her menstrual cycle.

PCO or PCOS (polycystic ovarian syndrome) Disorder noted by absence or abnormality of menstruation or irregular and abnormal menstruation, infertility, and often excess weight as well as excess body hair.

perimenopause A term used to describe hormonal fluctuations and their resultant complications prior to the time of normal menopause, as many as several years prior.

phytohormone Hormones found in plants, which may exert hormonal effects in the human body or even be identical to human hormone structure; phytosterol; among the differing types of phytohormones are isoflavones, lignans, sapogenins, and others.

PMS (premenstrual syndrome) One or more symptoms sometimes experienced in the days leading up to menstruation, such as abdominal pain, anxiety, headache, emotional lability, insomnia, and so on.

premature ovarian failure Loss of ovarian function in women under 40; also called POF; characterized by amenorrhea, low estrogen, and elevated FSH levels.

progesterone A female sex hormone secreted by the corpus luteum to prepare for the implantation of an egg into the uterus; during pregnancy, it is also secreted by the placenta in high levels to prevent rejection of the embryo or fetus; literally progestational; progesterone often accompanies estrogen in a hormone replacement therapy regimen.

progestin Synthetic analogs of progesterone with similar but not identical molecular structure; often used in hormone replacement therapy, where their widespread availability preceded the widespread availability of progesterone.

raloxifene A designer estrogen used to curb postmenopausal bone loss.

sapogenin A substance in plants that is the starting point in the synthesis of steroid hormones.

SERMs (selective estrogen receptor modulators) Chemicals that act on estrogen receptors in specific tissues to either potentiate or block the action of estrogens in the body.

tamoxifen A pill that interferes with the activity of estrogen and is used in addressing breast cancer.

testosterone A male sex hormone that is also seen in small quantities in females. In excess it is masculinizing. It is sometimes added to hormone replacement therapy to enhance libido, among other reasons.

traditional Chinese medicine (TCM) The centuries-old system of medicine from China, relying largely on combinations of herbal formulas and acupuncture to treat illness.

uterus Womb; the organ in a woman's body where an egg is implanted and where an embryo grows; the uterine lining is called the endometrium, which is sloughed off during menstruation.

vaginal atrophy Thinning and drying of vaginal tissues at menopause due to reduced levels of hormones.

vasomotor instability The possible cause of hot flashes; in vasomotor instability the blood vessels can dilate irregularly, leading to flushing, sweating, a feeling of heat, and associated symptoms.

xenohormone Literally those hormones that come from outside (*xeno-* means foreign); used to describe pollutants that exert hormonal effects or have a steroidal structure.

Resource Directory

Organizations and associations

American Board of Medical Specialties
(licensing board for specialists)
1007 Church St., Ste. 404
Evanston, Illinois 60201-5913
(847) 491-9091 or (800) 776-2378
Fax: (847) 328-3596
Web site: http://www.abms.org

American Board of Obstetrics & Gynecology
(licensing board)
2915 Vine St. Ste. 300
Dallas, TX 75204
(214) 871-1619
Fax: (214) 871-1943
Web site: http://www.abog.org
E-mail: info@abog.org

American Cancer Society
90 Park Ave.
New York, NY 10016
(212) 736-3030
Web site: www.cancer.org

American Heart Association
National Center
7272 Greenville Ave.
Dallas, Texas 75231
Heart and Stroke Information: (800) AHA-USA1
Women's Health Information: (888) MY-HEART
Web site: www.americanheart.org

American Society for Reproductive Medicine
1209 Montgomery Highway
Birmingham, AL 35216-2809
(205) 978-5000
Fax: (205) 978-5005
Web site: http://www.asrm.org
E-mail: asrm@asrm.org

National Osteoporosis Foundation
1150 17th St. NW, Ste. 500
Washington, DC 20036
(800) 223-9994
Web site: www.nof.org

National Women's Health Network
514 10th St. NW, Ste. 400
Washington, DC 20004
(202) 347-1140
Fax: (202) 347-1168

National Women's Health Resource Center, Inc.
(national clearinghouse for women's health
information)
120 Albany St., Ste. 820
New Brunswick, NJ 08901
Toll-Free (877) 98-NWHRC or (877) 986-9472
Main Number: (732) 828-8575
Fax: (732) 249-4671
Web site: www.healthywomen.org
E-Mail: NatlWHRC@aol.com

North America Menopause Society (NAMS)
PO Box 94527
Cleveland, OH 44101-4527
(216) 844-8748
Fax (216) 844-8708
Web site: www.menopause.org
E-mail: info@menopause.org

Internet resources

Newsgroups
alt.med.endometriosis
alt.support.menopause
alt.support.pco
misc.health.alternative
misc.health.infertility
sci.med.nutrition
sci.med.pharmacy
sci.med.obgyn
www.dejanews.com (for searching newsgroups)

Mailing lists
The Menopaus Mailing List
http://maelstrom.stjohns.edu/CGI/
wa.exe?SUBED1=menopaus&A=1
(to join the list)
http://www.howdyneighbor.com/menopaus/
index.html
(for more subscription information)

Web sites
Menopause
Menopause Online
http://www.menopause-online.com

MenoTimes
http://web.aimnet.com/~hyperion/meno/
menotimes.index.html

Midlife Passages
http://www.midlife-passages.com/page33.html

North American Menopause Society
http://www.menopause.org/

Infertility and pregnancy
Fertile Thoughts (infertility)
http://www.fertilethoughts.net

Midlife Pregnancy, Pregnancy, Childbirth Net
http://pregnancy.miningco.com/msubmidlife.htm

Women's Health Interactive Infertility Center
http://www.womens-health.com/InfertilityCenter/

Pharmacy and drugs
International Academy of Compounding
Pharmacists
http://www.compassnet.com/iacp

RxList: The Internet Drug Index
http://www.rxlist.com/

Medical conditions
Alzheimer's Prevention Foundation
http://www.brain-longevity.com/apf.html

American Cancer Society
http://www.cancer.org

American Heart Association
http://www.amhrt.org

Cancer News
http://www.cancernews.com

Gland Central (thyroid)
http://www.glandcentral.com

National Assn. for Incontinence
http://www.nafc.org

National Osteoporosis Foundation
http://www.nof.org

PCOSupport
The Polycystic Ovarian Syndrome Association
http://www.pcosupport.org

Premature Ovarian Failure (POF) Support Group
http://pofsupport.org

Thyroid Disease: The Mining Company
http://thyroid.miningco.com

Women's Cancer Network
http://www.wcn.org/

Clinical trials
CenterWatch Clinical Trials Listing Service
http://www.centerwatch.com

Women's health and general health
Achoo Internet Healthcare Directory
http://www.achoo.com

American Association of Clinical Endocrinologists
http://www.aace.com

American College of Obstetricians and
Gynecologists
http://www.acog.com

American Medical Association
http://www.ama-assn.org

American Society for Reproductive Medicine
http://www.asrm.com

Association of Reproductive Health Professionals
http://www.arhp.org

Bodymatters "Listening to Your Body"
http://bodymatters.com/bodymatters/
listening.html

HealthWorld Online
http://www.healthworld.com

MD Consult Clinical Information For Physicians
http://www.mdconsult.com

MedicineNet
http://www.medicinenet.com

Mediconsult.com Women's Health Medical
Information
http://www.mediconsult.com/women

National Women's Health Resource Center
http://www.healthywomen.org

Planned Parenthood
http://www.plannedparenthood.org

Web Directory: Doctor's Guide to the Internet
http://www.pslgroup.com/MENOPAUSE.HTM

Woman's Diagnostic Cyber—Women's Health
(Menopause)
http://www.wdxcyber.com

Women's Health (obgyn.net)
http://www.obgyn.net/women/conditions/
conditions.htm

Women's Health and Wellbeing WebRing
http://www.queendom.com/webring.html

Women's Health Hot Line
http://www.libov.com

Women's Health Interactive
http://www.womens-health.com

Alternative treatments for menopause
Acupuncture
http://www.acupuncture.com

National Center for Homeopathy
http://www.healthy.net/nch/index.html

National Qigong (Chi Kung) Association USA
http://www.nqa.org

Qigong Association of America
http://www.qi.org

Yoga for Menopause (Hot Flash Yoga)
http://www.hotflashyoga.com

Humor and human interest
Museum of Menstruation
http://www.mum.org

Medical searches
Medline Searches
http://www.ncbi.nlm.nih.gov/PubMed

Environmental issues
Endocrine Disruptors Research Initiative
http://www.epa.gov/endocrine

Responsible Care (Chemical Manufacturers Assn.)
http://www.cmahq.com/cmawebsite.nsf

Anti-aging
Anti-Aging Therapies
http://lef.org/anti-aging/index.html

Herbs, foods, and nutrition
Phytopharmacognosy Discussion Group Front Page
http://alpha2.mdx.ac.uk/www/pharm/noframes/
front.htm

The Herb Research Foundation
http://www.herbs.org

U.S. Soyfoods Directory
http://soyfoods.com

Recommended Reading List

Barnes, Broda O., and Lawrence Galton. *Hypothyroidism: The Unsuspected Illness.* Harper-Collins, 1976.

Cargill, Marie E. *Well Women: Healing the Female Body through Traditional Chinese Medicine.* Greenwood Publishing Group, Inc., 1998.

Crawford, Amanda McQuade. *The Herbal Menopause Book.* The Crossing Press, Inc., 1996.

Diamond, Jed. *Male Menopause: Sex & Survival in the Second Half of Life.* Sourcebooks, Inc., 1997.

Evans, Marie, Deborah Worksman, and Lysbeth Guillorn, (eds.). *The Noisy Passage; Menopause for the 21st Century.* Sourcebooks, Inc., 1997.

Gittleman, Ann Louise. *Before the Change: Taking Charge of Your Perimenopause.* Harper, 1998.

Greer, Germaine. *The Change: Women, Aging and the Menopause.* Fawcett Book Group, 1993.

Appendix C

Hadady, Letha, M.D. *Asian Health Secrets: The Complete Guide to Asian Herbal Medicine.* Random House Value Publishing, Inc., 1998.

Hill, Aubrey M. *Viropause/Andropause: The Male Menopause—Emotional & Physical Changes Midlife Men Experience.* New Horizon Press Publishers, Inc., 1993.

Horrigan, Bonnie. *Red Moon Passage: The Power and Wisdom of Menopause.* Random House Value Publishing, Inc., 1998.

Kamen, Betty. "Hormone Replacement Therapy Yes or No?: How to Make an Informed Decision About Estrogen, Progesterone, & Other Strategies for Dealing with PMS, Menopause." *Nutrition,* June 1995.

Komesaroff, Paul A. Philipa Rothfield, and Jeanne Daly (Editor). *Reinterpreting Menopause: Cultural and Philosophical Issues.* Routledge, 1996.

Lark, Susan M. *The Estrogen Decision Self Help Book.* Celestial Arts Publishing Company, 1995.

————. *Dr. Susan Lark's the Menopause Self Help Book: A Woman's Guide to Feeling Wonderful for the Second Half of Her Life.* Celestial Arts Publishing Company, 1992.

Laux, Marcus, and Christine Conrad. *Natural Woman, Natural Menopause.* HarperCollins Publishers, Inc., 1997.

Lee, John R., M.D., with Virginia Hopkins. *What Your Doctor May Not Tell You About Menopause: The Breakthrough Book on Natural Progesterone.* Warner Books. Inc., 1996.

Love, Susan M., and Karen Lindsey. *Dr. Susan Love's Hormone Book: Making Informed Choices About Menopause.* Random House, Inc., 1997.

Luchetti, Cathy, and Linda Hille. *The Hot Flash Cookbook.* Chronicle Books, 1997.

Northrup, Christiane. *Women's Bodies, Women's Wisdom: Creating Physical and Emotional Health and Healing.* Bantam Books, Inc., 1998.

Rako, Susan. *The Hormone of Desire: The Truth About Sexuality, Menopause, and Testosterone.* Harmony Books, 1996.

Sacks, Martha. *Menopaws: The Silent Meow.* Illustrated by Jack E. Davis. Ten Speed Press, 1995.

Shandler, Nina. *Estrogen: The Natural Way: Over 250 Easy and Delicious Recipes for Menopause.* Villard Books, 1997.

Sheehy, Gail. *The Silent Passage: Menopause.* Pocket Books, 1998.

Sheehy, Gail, and Joelle Delbourg. *New Passages: Mapping Your Life Across Time.* Ballantine Books, Inc., 1996.

Stringer, Nelson, H. *Uterine Fibroids: What Every Woman Needs to Know.* Physicians & Scientists Publishing Company, 1996.

Waterhouse, Debra. *Outsmarting the Midlife Fat Cell: Winning Weight Control Strategies for Women over 35 to Stay Fit Through Menopause.* Hyperion, 1998.

Wolf, Honora L. *Menopause, a Second Spring: Making a Smooth Transition with Traditional Chinese Medicine.* Blue Poppy, 1993.

The *Unofficial Guide*™ Reader Questionnaire

If you would like to express your opinion about coping with menopause or this guide, please complete this questionnaire and mail it to:

The *Unofficial Guide*™ Reader Questionnaire
Macmillan Lifestyle Group
1633 Broadway, floor 7
New York, NY 10019-6785

Gender: ___ M ___ F

Age: ___ Under 30 ___ 31–40 ___ 41–50
___ Over 50

Education: ___ High school ___ College
___ Graduate/Professional

What is your occupation?

_____

How did you hear about this guide?
___ Friend or relative
___ Newspaper, magazine, or Internet
___ Radio or TV
___ Recommended at bookstore
___ Recommended by librarian
___ Picked it up on my own
___ Familiar with the *Unofficial Guide*™ travel series

Did you go to the bookstore specifically for a book on menopause? Yes ___ No ___

Have you used any other *Unofficial Guides*™?
Yes ___ No ___

If Yes, which ones?

_____
_____
_____

What other book(s) on menopause have you purchased?

_____

_____

_____

Was this book:
___ more helpful than other(s)
___ less helpful than other(s)

Do you think this book was worth its price?
Yes ___   No ___

Did this book cover all topics related to menopause adequately?
Yes ___   No ___

Please explain your answer:

_____

_____

_____

Were there any specific sections in this book that were of particular help to you?   Yes ___   No ___

Please explain your answer:

_____

_____

_____

On a scale of 1 to 10, with 10 being the best rating, how would you rate this guide? ___

What other titles would you like to see published in the *Unofficial Guide*™ series?

_____

_____

Are *Unofficial Guides*™ readily available in your area?   Yes ___   No ___

Other comments:

_____

_____

_____

_____